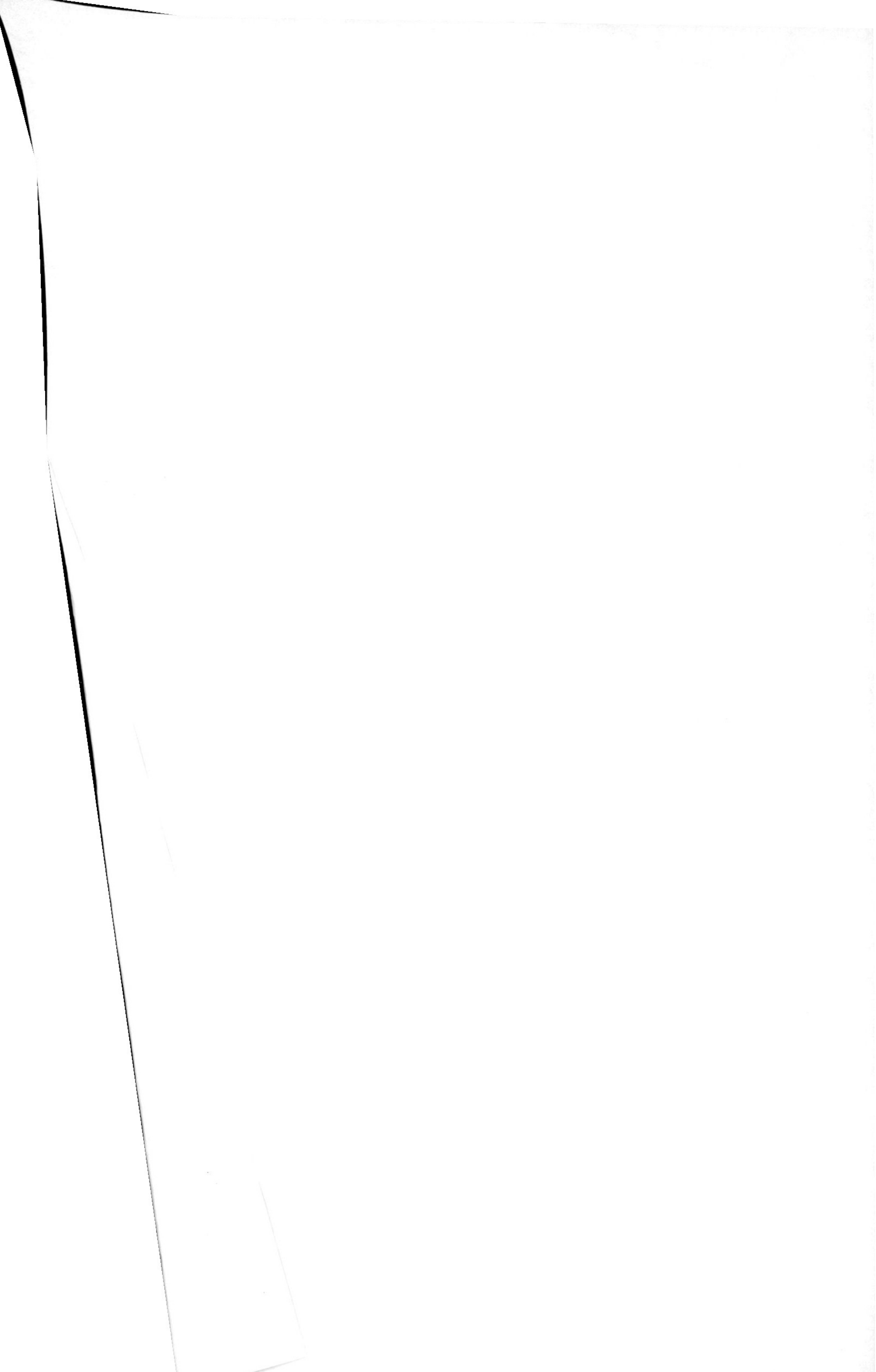

MARY CRAWFORD

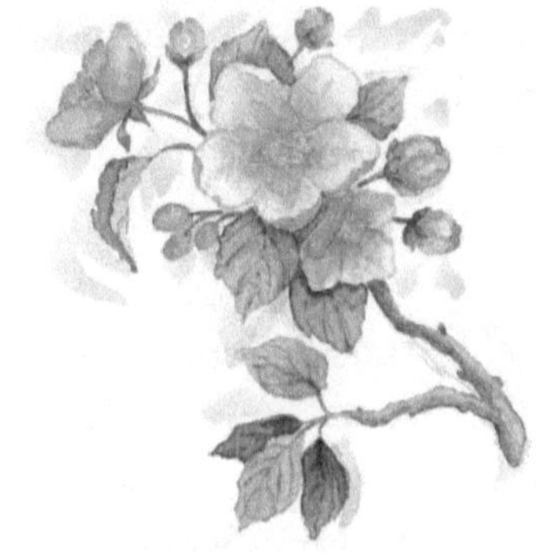

The Letter

HIDDEN BEAUTY BOOK 11

COPYRIGHT

HIDDEN BEAUTY SERIES

Until the Stars Fall from the Sky

So the Heart Can Dance

Joy and Tiers

Love Naturally

Love Seasoned

Love Claimed

If You Knew Me (and other silent musings)
(novella)

Jude's Song

The Price of Freedom (novella)

Paths Not Taken

Dreams Change (novella)

Heart Wish (100% charity release)

Tempting Fate

The Letter

The Power of Will

HIDDEN HEARTS SERIES

Identity of the Heart

Sheltered Hearts

Hearts of Jade

Port in the Storm (novella)

Love is More Than Skin Deep

Tough

Rectify

Pieces (a crossover novel)

Hearts Set Free

Freedom (a crossover novel)

The Long Road to Love (novella)

Love and Injustice (Protection Unit)

Out of Thin Air (Protection Unit)

Soul Scars (Protection Unit)

OTHER WORKS:

The Power of Dictation

Use Your Voice

An Everyday Guide to Scrivener 3 for Mac

Vision of the Heart

DEDICATION

To everyone who has faced down cancer
with ferocity and grim determination.
You have won more battles than most of us can fathom.

Kudos to the friends and family who provide the
invaluable support to help make that fight possible.

Chapter One

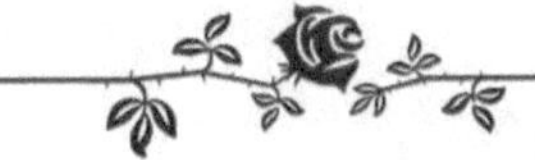

Rocco

As I wipe a wet cloth across my face, Jaxson comes into the locker room and sheds his scrubs. I nod at him. "Good afternoon, Doctor Shepherd."

"Call me Jax. My wife kicked our butts last weekend when we played pool. I think that earns you some special privileges."

"It's all right. When we're playing pool, I'll let the formal title slide. But, around here, you're still the doc and I'm still the guy who brings you the patients."

"Got news for you, Pierce. The patients would be much worse off if you and your fellow paramedics weren't so great at your jobs. Docs like us are grateful for all you do."

I stretch out my back and rub my temples. "I don't feel like such a hero today. We lost one twin in the MVA. Stupid drunk driver sheared off a third of the minivan."

"You did what you could. Because of you that mama still has one baby to hug tonight. I spent three hours rebuilding his leg. Recovery will take a while, but he's here."

I shake my head, trying to push away his words of praise. "You know me. I'd be happier if I could save them all."

Jaxson points down at his scrubs as he grabs a towel and heads to the shower. "Trust me — we all feel that way. Go home. You can't do any more here. I know you've had a crazy week. Get some sleep. You've earned it."

I scrub the heels of my hands over my eyes. "You're right. Maybe some sleep will put it into perspective."

⸻ ✦ ⸻

I kick the newspapers away from the front door as I grab a huge stack of mail from my mailbox. *Geez, when was the last time I checked my mail?* Jaxson is right. I need to take some down time. One day bleeds into the next. As soon as I throw my mail on the kitchen table and set my food down, my cat jumps from the floor to my shoulder. Fortunately, this time Chevy makes it on his first shot. Chevy isn't known for his grace. He meows loudly in my ear.

"I hear ya buddy. I'm starving too." I murmur as I grab a can of cat food from the pantry and pop it open. Chevy hops down as I place it on the floor beside his water dish.

Exhausted, I slump down in the nearest chair. I take a sip of my Coke and unwrap my sandwich. After I take a bite and set it down, the logo on a piece of my mail catches my eye. That's weird. They said it would take a couple of months for my raise to come through after I qualified for the next pay grade.

Curious, I rip open the large envelope and skim the contents. I blink, shake my head and read it again. None of this is making any sense. It's not from payroll. This is from radiology. I double check. It's addressed to me — Rocco A. Pierce. It even has my phone number — but the letter refers a mammogram. The patient's name is Mallory F. Yoshida. It would seem I'm listed as her spouse.

One problem. I've never been married.

Chevy looks up at me with a confused expression on his face as he tries to make sense of my agitated movements. I flip the large envelope over and dump out the rest of the contents. To my surprise, a disk lands on my kitchen table. With trepidation, I scoop it up and walk over to my desk and boot up my computer. As I wait for it to finish, I read the radiology report I found folded in the cardboard with the disc. I cringe when I reach the conclusion. I'm no doctor, but I am familiar with medical terminology. Whoever Mallory Yoshida is, she is in for the fight of her life. I press eject on the CD drive on my computer and place the CD on the tray.

Even though I see women's torsos frequently in my job, it seems a little voyeuristic to be looking at a stranger's mammogram. When the images appear in front of me, I'm surprised. I don't know exactly what I was expecting. I suppose with a BI-RADS score of five, I figured the cancer would be obvious. Using my touchscreen, I zoom in a bit closer. Eventually, I find a white area on what would be the underside of her left breast.

I blow the air out of my lungs and draw in a quick breath. Part of me was hoping all this was a weird clerical error. Unfortunately, it looks like the radiologist had a good reason for being ninety-five percent sure this woman has breast cancer.

As sad as that is, it still doesn't answer one fundamental question: what does it all have to do with me?

A feeling of dread passes over me. I unclip my cell phone from my belt loop. Swallowing hard, I dial my mom's number.

"Rocco? Is that you? It's loud in here. Your father is watching Wheel of Fortune again. He solved the last puzzle when none of the contestants knew what it was. I keep telling him he ought to try out for the show."

"He probably should. Listen, I won't keep you long … I need to know, when was the last time you had a mammogram?"

"Rocco! You don't ask a lady such a thing! I thought I raised you with better manners. I think being a paramedic has gone to your head. You think you can ask anybody anything."

"Totally true. But I've got a reason for asking —"

"What possible reason could you have?"

"Mom, I can't even begin to explain. Could you just tell me?"

"Well, if you must know — I always have them around my birthday."

"Did you get your results back? Are you okay?"

"Of course I did. I would've told you if something was amiss."

"Okay, thank you for telling me. I need to go, it's been a long week. I'm completely beat."

"I can tell. Rocco, if you've been drinking, knock it off. You were always a rather strange child, but this conversation is over the top, even for you."

"Mom! I'm stone cold sober, I promise. There's a bunch of stuff going on I don't even understand right now."

My mother makes a clicking sound with her tongue. "I don't know if I find your explanation comforting or if it scares me even more."

"Good night, Mom. Love you."

"Love you, sleep tight. Try not to work so hard."

CHAPTER TWO

MALLORY

GROANING, I PLACE ONE last zucchini in the overflowing basket of produce. Edna grins cheekily at me as she offers me her cane. "You need this, sweetie?"

"I might." I balance gingerly as I stand up. "I twisted my knee funny on my stair workout."

Edna shakes her head at me. "Never did see the purpose of you running up and down those bleachers anyway. Why would you go and run someplace you don't have to — and then do it over and over again?"

I pick up the basket and walk toward Edna's house. "Oh, I don't know. Maybe it's because I'd like to fit through my doorway after my next-door neighbor spoils me with world-class goodies."

"Oh come now, Miss Mallory, I don't spoil you so much."

"Yes, you do Edna. I don't know what I would do without you. The only thing I have in my refrigerator is milk for my cereal in the morning and a little coffee creamer. Everything else is so old it should probably be thrown out. You are far better to me than I ever deserve. You've practically adopted me."

"Don't be silly. I know you have parents. It's not your fault they are too busy to notice what a lovely young woman you are. Besides, they live all the way across the United States. You need someone close. Now, let's talk about your knee. You know, I have a perfectly nice orthopedic doctor. He's cute too."

It's a good thing I am busy scrubbing potatoes and Edna can't see my eye roll — but I'm sure she knows my expressions by now. I turn around to face her. "How many times do I have to tell you? I'm too busy for a boyfriend. You do *not* have to fix me up. Besides, the doctor type wouldn't be interested in a crime reporter for a webzine."

"Honey, I'm not even sure I know what that is. But all I can say is don't sell yourself short. When I met my Gordon, he was working on the space shuttle project and I was a simple hairdresser. He fell in love with me just the same. I tell people love isn't like rocket science." Edna giggles. She sobers as tears gather in her eyes. "I miss him so much. Getting old sucks!"

I take a package of frozen peas out of Edna's freezer and ice my knee as I limp over to her breakfast bar. "Tell me about it — and I'm only twenty-seven."

"No, you don't understand. My doctor wants me to go do a test where they stick a camera up my rectum! Can you imagine? Will you go with me? You can have it done first, like you did the mammogram —"

"Oh Edna …" I hedge. "I appreciate the offer, but I don't need a colonoscopy. I only did the mammogram because you were petrified to do it. I won't need to do a colonoscopy for another twenty-some years. Besides, you'll be asleep through the process."

"But you went with me to the dentist to check him out —" she argues stubbornly.

"I did — but that was different. I actually needed my teeth cleaned."

"And you went to the eye doctor."

I wince. "True enough, although I still can't figure out why I was there. The medical staff told me you go to Doctor Moore all the time to have your glaucoma checked and you have for years. According to them, you treat him like your grandson."

"He is one of the sweetest men I know. I just wanted the two of you to meet. He is a hottie, isn't he?"

"*Argh!* Edna, I love you, you know that? But, you cannot keep coercing me into medical appointments to introduce me to cute doctors. I don't know if you know — but I work for a small company which doesn't offer health insurance. Your matchmaking strategy is making me go broke!"

"What do you mean? Aren't those visits free?"

"No, why would they be?"

"Well, I figured since I referred you and it was your first time, you would get a complimentary visit or something."

"Sorry to tell you but medicine has changed. These days, you get charged for a Band-Aid."

"I'm so sorry Miss Mallory. I didn't mean to put you out. The honest truth is my world hasn't been the same since our daughter died. She's been gone longer than you've been alive. But I still miss her every single day. I don't want a nice girl like you to end up with the kind of creep who killed my baby girl."

I stand up and walk around to give Edna a hug. "Don't worry. I'm in no hurry to be in a relationship. In my line of work, I see a million ways how it can all go wrong."

Edna sighs. "I wish my Gordon was around. I'd feel better if he could protect you from the riff-raff."

"Something tells me not much riff-raff would get by you either."

Edna picks up her cane. "That's true. I have this, and Lulu has a sense about men." She points to her Yorkie curled into a ball sleeping front of the fireplace.

Shedding my corporate jacket, I head over to my assistant's desk. "Okay, Andre, I'm finally here. What did I miss while I was held captive in the world's longest staff meeting?"

"What were you guys doing in there? Holding a séance?"

"Practically. There were four experts arguing over how net neutrality will impact our advertisers."

"What was the verdict?"

"It's grim. No one can seem to agree on how grim. I'm just going to put my head down and do my job. Maybe someday I'll wake up and not have a job and have to figure out what to do, but until then, I'll just do what I do."

"Your job just got a little more exciting. I heard from one of my CIs in law enforcement. You know the case we've been following —"

I draw in a sharp breath. "Oh my gosh! They got back to you about the basketball player?"

"The very one," Andre answers smugly.

"How in the world did you get so lucky? I've been chasing that lead for months."

Andre clears his throat. "Sometimes, my less than savory past gives me connections you just don't have."

"I guess. So, what did you find out?"

"The DNA is not a match."

"They couldn't figure that out before Marshall Todd spent seven and a half years in jail?"

"Depends on who you talk to. Some people swear there wasn't DNA to test. Other people say the DNA was there all along, but it was simply suppressed because it didn't match the suspect they wanted to prosecute."

"Wow! Just wow. Anybody willing to go on record?"

Andre shrugs. "Perhaps … if we tread carefully."

"Does anybody else know about this? What about the accuser? Where is she in this saga? Is she willing to talk?" I pepper Andre with questions as fast as they fly into my consciousness.

"I don't know if this is a scoop. Knowing my sources, I wouldn't be surprised if she is ready to talk. You should probably interview her. I closely resemble the guy she tried to frame. I don't think she's gonna want to talk to me."

"Good point. Besides, I seem to have one of those faces that encourages people to tell me their entire life story, maybe it'll work on Sheila Taylor."

"I think once she figures out how much you care about this story, she'll want to talk to you."

"I hope so. Her story could put a whole new spin on things. I've been researching this story for years and her side of it has never made any sense."

Andre nods. "You know, I've never figured that out. I mean, I know why I want to see Marshall Todd get justice. It's one of those 'but for the grace of God go I' stories for me, but why are you so passionate about it?"

I stretch out a kink in my neck as I ponder how to answer Andre's question. "I went into journalism because I wanted to help make the world make sense. After my friend Juliette was attacked, I realized how messed up the world of criminal justice is. The case of Marshall Todd is the most egregious case of injustice I have ever seen. The more I look into it, the worse it gets. I want to find out how the case went off the rails and see if I can do anything to fix what went wrong. I firmly believe Marshall Todd was wrongly convicted. I think Sheila Taylor has some of the answers I'm looking for."

"I think you're right. Let me see what I can do about arranging an interview for you."

"I guess I better start prepping for the interview of my life. Who knows? I might get lucky. Who am I kidding? What makes me think she'd have any interest in talking to me? I'm just a nobody from a no-name online newspaper. She's probably never even heard of me."

"Don't let where you work define your skills as a journalist. You simply had the bad luck to have the world's worst boss your first job right out of college. It was the luck of the draw. It's only a temporary setback on your career path."

"Yeah, that's what I keep telling myself. But the whole sexual harassment mess was a while ago now and my career is still stuck in neutral. So, what does that say about me?"

"Primarily, it says you're not willing to move to a bigger market because you like living in the middle of nowhere and picking tomatoes from your neighbor's garden."

I grin. "You're not wrong. I'd just like to figure out how to win a Pulitzer from here."

Chapter Three

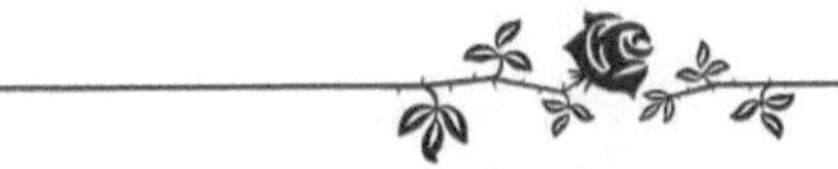

Rocco

I GRIT MY TEETH and try again. Glancing down at her name tag I say as calmly as I can, "No, Melodi, I'm not trying to get the information in Ms. Yoshida's medical records, I'm trying to give it back to you."

"Why would you try to give us back your wife's medical records?"

"As I have explained four times, Ms. Yoshida is not my wife. No one has ever been my wife."

Melodi points to the letter. "It says right here she's your wife."

"I know what it says — but that's not the case. I think I would know if I've ever been married."

"Why aren't you married? A cute guy like you? There must be something wrong with you. Are you some loser who can't keep a job?"

"No! I'm a paramedic!"

"Ooh how sexy!" she coos as she reaches out to run her hand through my close-cropped hair.

I back away. "Being a paramedic is lots of things. Sexy is not one of them."

"I read lots of those steamy romance novels. They have firefighters and paramedics all the time. The things their bodies can do are incredible. Their muscles have muscles. I bet you're like that. I'd let you give me mouth-to-mouth anytime. It would be totally hot."

I clear my throat. "I've never actually read one of those books — but it sounds like they use more than a little artistic interpretation. Can we just try to figure out how to get Ms. Yoshida her medical records, please?"

Her bottom lip pops out, and she looks a tad dejected. "So, you're telling me not only are you not married to this lady, you don't even know her?"

I nod vigorously. "Exactly!"

"So how come your name is on her medical records?"

"I have no earthly clue. I was hoping you could tell me."

Melodi takes a few moments to study her computer screen. She goes to another computer and pulls up a different screen. Tucking a pen behind her ear, she walks back and forth between the two computers. Finally she looks up at me. "Where did you say you got these?"

"Two days ago, I checked my mailbox and an envelope was in there. I hadn't checked my mail in a few days because I've been working back-to-back shifts and I was exhausted. It could have been there for several days."

Melodi pulls the envelope from the stack of papers. "This is the envelope it came in?"

"It is."

"That's weird. We changed our stationary a couple of months ago. We have a new logo now."

"So? Maybe they were using up old stock."

"We were told to destroy the old stuff because they wanted a unified brand."

"Seems wasteful … but okay —"

"You've got a big problem. Mallory Yoshida does not exist."

"What do you *mean* she doesn't exist? This mammogram is from this hospital. This letter is issued from this radiology department. That's your return address on the letter."

"All of that might be true — but Mallory Yoshida does not exist."

"Melodi, use your common sense. I looked at the disc. Those are someone's breasts on the mammogram — someone who got a five on the BI-RADS scale. The radiologist is ninety-five percent sure she's got cancer. Those are crappy odds if she goes untreated."

"You have no idea how much I wish I could help you. I'd love for you to owe me a favor. But if she doesn't exist in our system, there's nothing I can do."

"So that's it?"

"Well, look on the bright side. They were wrong about her being married to you — maybe they're wrong about everything else too," Melodi suggests as she shrugs.

"Under the circumstances, I pray you're right."

⚊⚊⚊●⚊⚊⚊

"Jaxson, if you're finished laughing your butt off … I'm not kidding. Swing by my house when we're done, and I'll show you."

"Rocco, if this chick is real, don't open yourself up to any more HIPPA violations by sharing."

I scrub my hand down my face. "Oh man, I wasn't even thinking about this through the prism of privacy laws. I was more worried about getting her the information."

"Records says she doesn't exist?"

"Not a trace. Radiology can't find her either."

"What about the radiologist who read the x-rays?"

"He read the mammogram but has no memory of the specific case. He was zero help. This whole thing is hurting my professional reputation. People are questioning my sanity."

"If they're just now starting to question your sanity, they haven't known you long enough," Jaxson quips.

"Hilarious! Not necessarily wrong, but funny nonetheless."

"Okay, so no one can find your mysterious Mallory Yoshida. What if she really is an imaginary patient?"

"Come again? I saw the films, remember?"

"You saw films. But you didn't necessarily see *her* films. They could've been manipulated like everything else in her file."

"I'm not sure I follow," I admit.

"In medical school when we were learning clinical skills, we had imaginary patients with imaginary charts. We had to treat their imaginary illnesses and review their imaginary documentation and imaginary tests to come up with our imaginary diagnosis. You may have run across a sophisticated version of that in the real world."

"How would these files get mixed in with real medical records?"

"I have no idea. I suppose it could be a crazy medical school prank or something. But it would explain how a patient could disappear off the planet."

"In theory, I guess you're right. That would be the most logical explanation. Somehow, I can't shake the feeling there's more to it."

"Rocco, for the sake of your career, stick to the facts you know. Save your emotions for when you play video games."

From the corner of the room, I hear Donda, Jaxson's wife, snort with laughter. "Are you kidding me, Jax? What happened to you? When did you become such a fuddy-duddy?" She nods and laughs. "I'm here today because this guy followed a wild hunch and drove miles out of his way just to cross paths with me, remember? Jax didn't just do it for one day; he followed me for weeks before we actually met."

I raise an eyebrow and look at Jaxson. "True?"

He chuckles. "Busted."

"He also followed his gut when he diagnosed me with endocarditis. Jax didn't follow any prescribed protocol. He just acted and saved my life."

Donda puts her drawing tablet down, walks over to the sideboard, and grabs a sticky pad. She pulls a number up in her phone and writes it down. As she squats down next to me, she looks me in the eyes. "I'm not telling you what to do. But, if you decide to look for this woman, Tobias Payne can work miracles. He works for a company called Identity Bank West. He was once missing, so he knows what it means to be found."

Something about Donda's words touches the core of the issue for me. What if it's already too late? The mammogram was done a couple months ago. I don't know enough about breast cancer to know how aggressive her tumor might be. Despite the hospital's insistence Mallory does not exist and Jaxson's theory that she might be a fictitious patient used only for educational purposes, I know I must find Mallory Yoshida.

———————◆———————

"To be honest, when you told me you had someone you needed me to find, I figured it would be a challenge." Toby says as he hands me a file. "I totally didn't expect it to be somebody I already follow on social media."

"Seriously?" I ask, as I try to remember to close my gaping mouth.

"Yeah, Mallory Yoshida has a righteous crime column. She's like a crusader against bad guys. She's not exactly hidden."

"Are you sure it's the same person?"

"Well, as certain as I can be without talking to her. The demographics match — except for the fact that she's not married to you, of course. A couple of years ago, her office threw her a quadranscentennial party."

"A what?"

Toby laughs at my confusion. "I know. I had to look it up too. It means twenty-fifth anniversary. She works at an avant-garde online newspaper. They're a little quirky. I guess it's just another name for her twenty-fifth birthday."

"Oh wow! So, it actually could be her?"

"The part I don't get is why somebody her age would be getting a test like that. Isn't it something somebody like my mom would do?" Toby asks as he turns slightly red.

"Usually. But, maybe Mallory has a family history of cancer or something. I hope not. Cancer sucks." I run my finger over the embossed logo on the file as I look up at Toby. "Okay, break the bad news to me. You told me she works at this quirky dot com company. Where do I have to go to track her down, New York or Silicon Valley?"

Toby snickers. "Nothing so exotic. According to my sources, Mallory Yoshida lives in Sublimity. *Word Soup PNW* is headquartered in Salem.

I lean back in my chair and blow out the breath I didn't realize I was holding. "I don't know what to say. Great job, Toby. Thanks! Now I have to figure out what to do. I thought this process would take a long time and I'd have time to come up with a plan."

"I wish I had some great advice for you — I just don't. I'm sorry, dude. She'll probably hate you. There's not much you can do about that. Even if you had great news to tell her, you're still disrupting her world. Let's face it, no matter how you dress it up, you don't have great news. This is one of those situations where you go in and try to do as little damage as possible. I don't think you get to be the hero here."

I stand up and shake Toby's hand. "Thanks for the reality check. You're right. I'll be doing well to just minimize the damage in my wake. I'll be in touch if I need anything else."

"I know this sounds stupid, but you seem to be kinda like me. Remember, you didn't cause those cancer cells to grow. You're just trying to make the problem better. You're not responsible for Mallory's well-being."

I glance at him in wide-eyed surprise. "Apparently, Mallory's background isn't the only one you researched thoroughly."

Toby shrugs. "At Identity Bank West, we can't be too careful. Before we hand over private, personal information, we need to understand where it's going."

"Understood. Thank you for trusting me."

"I know this will be hard. But the world needs more stand-up guys like you. Good luck."

Chapter Four

Mallory

Andre compulsively picks up the sandwich wrapper and the discarded bag of chips from around my computer and throws them in the trash. "Did you even step away from your computer all day? Go stretch your legs!" He shakes his head at me. When he sees a smear of mustard on my keyboard, he scowls at me. "What have I told you about eating at your desk?" He removes an antibacterial wipe from my bottom desk drawer. He looks back up at me. "I wasn't kidding. Go! We'll talk when you get back."

People in the office are standing up to look over their cubicles at the ruckus he is creating. With as much dignity as I can muster, I stand up and walk out of my office area. Granted, I've worked my way up to a corner cubicle, but it's still a cubicle.

After a short stop at the facilities, I walk to my favorite coffee shop. I stand quietly behind two college interns we hired a couple weeks ago. The brunette turns to the redhead and says, "I don't know why Andre drools all over her. He's the cutest guy in the place. It's pathetic to see."

The redhead shrugs. "Beats me. Maybe he's trying to sleep his way to the top. He is her assistant. She has a regular byline. I don't think she's so pretty — you know, she's got the whole Asian thing and some guys like exotic, but sometimes you gotta take one for the team — you know what I mean?"

"Yeah, I tried to get his attention. I figured it would help my grade if I could get in good with the boss. He completely blew me off." She throws her thick mane of brown hair over her shoulder. "Guys don't usually do that."

I clear my throat behind them. I get more than a little satisfaction when they both jump and look like they've seen a ghost. "Maybe it's because Andre is engaged. But, even before then, he wasn't the type to pick up partners simply to advance his career. If you're looking for that kind of workplace, *Word Soup* isn't it. Maybe you guys should find an internship more suited to your expectations."

The redhead becomes so pale she looks like she might pass out. "Oh no! Please don't make us leave. This is our second placement. It's our last chance. They'll kick us out of the class if we don't complete it this time."

The brunette joins her plea. "It's true. My dad will kill me if I don't graduate."

"What was your infraction at the last job?"

The redhead hangs her head. "Gossiping too much. They accused us of unprofessional behavior inconsistent with the tenets of journalism."

I raise an eyebrow. "I take it the lesson didn't stick."

The brunette huffs. "We thought we were alone."

I roll my eyes. "In the middle of a busy coffee shop? Hardly. Word to the wise. Everybody around here likes and respects Andre. You know why? He treats everyone like gold. Don't try to trash his reputation. The only person you make look small is you."

Tears gather in the eyes of the redhead. "Sorry," she mumbles.

"What are you planning to do to us?"

"Unfortunately for you, you started building your professional reputation the day you started school. That includes your internships — for better or worse. You are in the driver's seat. You guys can choose to act like you're in junior high school or you can comport yourself like the professionals you say you want to be. The choice is yours."

The couple ahead of them in line leaves and the barista is waiting for their order. They look at me as if asking for permission to proceed. I nod and gesture toward the counter. The brunette stammers her order and tells the woman her name is Leah. The redhead gives her order in a voice so soft, the barista has to lean over the counter to hear. When she announces her name, I smile. I can't believe I forgot. Harmony is such a beautiful name.

When they turn around, they have to face me again. They are clutching their coffee so tight I'm amazed the cups don't collapse.

"Now what?" Harmony whispers.

"Andre has a huge archiving project he needs help with."

"But, that's not —" Leah starts to protest.

"Thank you. We'll get right on that," Harmony says as she nudges Leah with her elbow and shoots her an annoyed look.

———— ● ————

"Geez, I thought you were taking a coffee break. I didn't realize you were taking a mini vacation," comments Andre as he looks at his watch.

I blow my bangs out of my eyes as I set a large cup of coffee down on his desk. I take a sip of my drink before I answer, "I had to deal with a little something which popped up."

He narrows his eyes at me over the top of his coffee cup. "Anything major?"

"Could've been. Hope it's not now. We'll see."

I lock my purse in the cupboard behind my desk and flop down in my ergonomic chair. It's my favorite luxury in this little cubicle of mine. The rest of my cubicle is a bit of a disaster area. There are research files stacked everywhere. Andre has a system to keep me organized — but I have several stories in various stages of completion and notes and background information piled up on every surface available. Andre insists on surrounding me with healthy greenery and plants. Fortunately for me, he has the skills to keep them alive. I love flowers and plants, but I am not gifted in keeping them healthy.

"What's been keeping you so busy you haven't even checked your email messages from me?"

I rub my temples. "I've been reading the transcripts from Marshall Todd's trial. It's a weird experience knowing what we know now. I lurch from bone numbing boredom to white-hot rage."

"Have you gotten to Sheila's testimony yet?"

"I just started on direct. I wish it was on videotape. Sheila was inconsistent and jumpy in her testimony. I guess it must've seemed like she was coached because the court reporter even referred to her looking out into the audience like she was waiting for an answer a couple of times."

Andre pulls the file away from me and turns it around so he can read it. "Are you serious?"

I pick up a pen and point out the parenthetical comment where the court reporter refers to the noise in the gallery and Sheila's subsequent answer.

"Wow! I'm surprised the judge let it stand."

"It's like one of a thousand things which happened to make this trial incredibly unfair to Marshall. I wish I could've been there to see who the mysterious guy in the audience was. Was it an attorney? Was it Sheila's boyfriend? Now we'll never know. This is so frustrating."

"We might never know *if* Sheila doesn't talk to you. That's what all this prep is about, remember? You have been my boss for years now. There's one thing I know about you. You look all unassuming and mouse-like. But you are one of the most formidable people I know. If anyone can persuade Sheila to talk, it's you. Not only will you get her to talk, she'll spill her secrets like you're her long-lost best friend. She'll tell you thoughts she didn't even know she had. You've got this Mal."

"You think so?"

"I know so. I could go work for one of the big news stations in Portland — trust me they've asked. But nobody is a better reporter than you. I stick with the best."

"Thank you, Andre. I don't know what I did to

deserve you. I guess I better get back to earning that title," I say as I put my earbuds back in.

Andre reaches out to stop me. "Not so fast. We have to talk. I don't send you emails because I'm bored."

I take my earbuds out and lean back in my chair as I click on my in-box. "Okay, lay it on me. Did I suddenly win the lottery? Has my dad forgiven me for not becoming a dentist?"

"Not that I know of — but those things would be great. Does the name Rocco Pierce mean anything to you?"

I pull up my phone contacts and nothing comes up. I shake my head. "No, should it?"

Andre looks dejected. "Crap! He's been so persistent; I was hoping he was a contact for Marshall's story. His name doesn't sound familiar to me either."

"What do you mean?" I ask as I sit up and grab a pad of paper.

"Well, I sent him the usual automated string of letters we send fans in case he is merely a crime story junkie. Usually, that appeases most people."

"But not him? Do we have a background check on this guy?"

Andre nods. "He works out of Yamhill County. He's a paramedic. By all accounts, he's a normal dude with heroic tendencies. He received an award for volunteer work with homeless kids."

"Okay, sounds good to me. What set off your protective big brother radar? Does he look like a serial killer or something?"

"Oh honey, he is a fine specimen of a man. He gives

my fiancé, Philip, a run for his money. He has very kind eyes — it's not his looks that bother me. I'm worried because he doesn't really want to correspond with me. He insists he needs to talk to you about a letter. When I asked him what the letter was regarding, he told me it was personal and confidential."

"That's strange."

"You got any unsettled scores with old boyfriends?"

I click my pen for a couple seconds before I shrug. "You know about the only controversial situations I was ever involved in. As far as I know, one guy is still the head of a news division and the other guy is cooling his jets in jail."

A sympathetic look crosses Andre's face. "How is Juliette doing?"

"Better since she made it through JR's first parole hearing. The creep pretty much screwed himself for future parole hearings when he told the parole board he would never apologize for hitting her so hard she lost the hearing in her left ear. He tried to intimidate me too — but I glared right back. I can't believe I was ever his friend."

"Like I said, you are one of the most quietly intimidating people I know. You may be a tiny waif, but you're tough. Your testimony helped put him away. He destroyed Juliette's memories of that day, so she needed you. I wonder if this Rocco Pierce is related to her case?"

I frown. "I hope not. I want to put the whole incident behind me. My best friend didn't deserve to become partially deaf and have a permanent brain injury because my other former friend became jealous of her boyfriend." I try to shake off my dark thoughts. "Andre, what do you think I should do about this?"

Andre walks over to his desk and picks up a folder. He brings it over to me and places it in my hands. "Take this and read it. It's all the correspondence I've had with the guy. It includes the background information Loralee was able to dig up on him. It won't tell you everything, but maybe it'll give you a sense of him. I can tell you he seems determined to talk to you. Maybe there's a good reason."

A chill goes up my spine as I take the file from Andre. A sense of foreboding overtakes me. Suddenly it feels like this is the most important decision I'll ever make.

Chapter Five

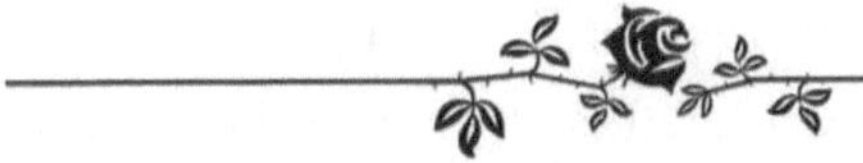

Rocco

"Mom, I can't believe you went to all this effort. You know homemade macaroni and cheese is my favorite. It's not even my birthday or anything. It's a random Saturday afternoon."

"Nonsense, you know your dad likes it is much as you do. We're just happy you're here. It seems you've been working a lot of weekends lately. Your dad was wondering if you'd ever be free to go fishing again."

"We've had a couple of new hires recently. Things should slow down a bit soon."

My phone vibrates in my pocket. I hold my finger up to my mom. "I'm sorry, I have to get this."

My parents' voices fade in the background as I check my messages. My mom turns to my dad. "Remember when we didn't answer the phone during meals, Rick?"

"The technology is different these days, Veronica. Our son has an important job."

My eyes widen as I read the message. I've waited weeks for this to happen. Now that it has, I'm not sure what to say.

"Rocco?" my mom interrupts my panicked musings. "What's wrong?"

"Nothing," I started to answer and then abruptly change my mind. "No, that's not right. Everything is wrong with this situation. I have to figure out how to tell a perfect stranger they may die."

My dad sets down his fork. "That's tragic, son. But, don't you do something similar nearly every day?"

"I suppose so. But for some reason this feels so much different. This woman is simply going about her life and I'm about to pull the rug out from under her and make everything she thought she knew about her life seem like a lie."

My mom draws in a sharp breath. "Oh my heavens, Rocco. Does this have anything to do with that very strange conversation we had several weeks ago?"

Wearily, I nod.

My mom takes a napkin and wipes the corner of her eye. "Life is so unfair."

"Mom, I have no idea what to say." The enormity of the task suddenly catches up with me.

"The best you can do is be as honest as you can, while being compassionate. You can't make the truth hurt any less."

"Thanks." I set my napkin down on the table. "I need to go deal with this. I love you guys."

"We love you too. We'll leave the door open for you in case you need a shoulder to cry on when you're done."

"Depending on how it goes, you may have a deal."

———————●———————

I glance around the room my mom calls the den. It's funny she calls it that, because it still bears a strong resemblance to my childhood room. The only concession she's made to the reality that I've long ago grown up and moved away is a new roll-top desk and the appearance of her favorite sewing machine. I walk over to my ancient stereo and pop in my favorite Bob Seger CD as I try to calm my nerves.

Finally, I calm down enough to sit down in the over-sized leather chair and reread the text message I received earlier.

"What's so important that you have to harass my assistant, but you can't talk about in a text message?"

"It's difficult to explain," I text back carefully. "I need to speak to you in person."

"I'm sorry. I cover the crime beat. For safety reasons, I don't meet with fans. I'm sure you understand," came her quick reply.

"I'm sure you are a powerful writer, but this isn't about your job. It's much more personal."

"You know, you're not helping your case here."

"I understand. I'm trying to be honest. I can give you the name of my supervisor at work. I'm not a bad guy. This is just something I can't explain through a text message."

"Have we ever met before?"

"I don't think so," I cringe as I type those words. I can feel any hope of meeting Mallory slip through my fingers.

"Why do you feel this is so important if you don't even know me?"

"Because it's the right thing to do," I answer candidly.

"Kinda hung up on the whole right and wrong thing, aren't you?" she responds with an eye roll emoji. "Even if I asked to talk to your boss, how do I know it's not just one of your drinking buddies?"

"I don't have many of those. I'm a paramedic. It's bad form to show up to a call drunk."

For several minutes, my phone is so silent; I'm afraid maybe my battery went dead. I shake my phone and hit the volume button just to confirm it still works. I take a long drink of my coffee and doodle aimlessly on a tablet of paper. I'm almost afraid to breathe for fear I'll miss her text message.

My phone beeps. I hold my breath as I check my phone. "Okay, let's say I believe you. Is it okay if my friends are nearby when we meet? I would feel safer."

"Understood. Where do you want to meet?"

"Do you know where the carousel is at the Riverfront Park in Salem?"

"I do. I've taken my friend's daughter there often. I can meet you there in about an hour."

"Sounds good. You better not be pulling some weird, sick joke on me," she warns.

Sighing, I text back, "Mallory, you have no idea how much I wish I was. I'll see you in an hour. Wait … how will I know it's you?"

"I've got black hair and I'll be wearing a bright red jacket," she responds. "I might be short, but I'm hard to miss," she texts a smiley face. "I'll be sitting on the park benches by the gazebo."

"I look like a typical Oregon hipster. I'm wearing a Portland Timbers hockey jersey today. I am a tall guy with a blue eyes."

"This feels like we're meeting for an over-the-top blind date or something," Mallory texts.

"I wish it were that simple."

"You have my Spidey senses as a reporter going crazy."

"Like I said, it's complicated — I'll explain more later. I just hope you don't hate me when I'm done."

"Are you trying to talk yourself into a meeting or out of one? You're scaring me!"

"Mallory, I mean you no harm. Your friends can stay right by your side, I promise — I just need to talk to you."

"Hurry! Now I don't want to wait to hear what you have to say. I'm dying of curiosity."

"Okay, I'll be there as soon as I can."

As I put on my coat and stick my phone in my pocket, I wonder if there is a polite way to tell someone they may be dying of more than simple curiosity.

* * *

My stomach turns slightly as I stride toward the gazebo. Mallory's back is to me when I first approach. All the fancy words I rehearsed on the way over fly out of my head when she turns to watch my arrival. I try to read her expression as her friend elbows her and leans over and whispers something in her ear. All I can think about is how impossibly young she looks. I guess cancer doesn't care.

She brushes her jet-black hair out of her eyes after a gust of wind hits it. She squints and looks up at me. "You must be Rocco. I'm Mallory." She extends her hand for me to shake and then gestures over at the guy standing protectively next to her. "This is Andre."

I politely shake her hand and attempt to hide my surprise as a weird warm shock seems to pass between the two of us. Mallory seems as startled as I am. She clears her throat and pulls her hand back. Andre is watching the interaction with fascination as he shakes my hand. "What's with the cloak and dagger approach? Do you have something on the Marshall Todd case?"

My eyes widen. "No! I wish. My older brother played ball against him in high school. Remy never believed he was guilty."

"So, why are you here? I'm certain I would remember you if we'd ever met." Mallory looks ready to jump out of her skin as she carefully studies me.

I quickly glance over at Andre as I decide how much to disclose. The way he's holding her protectively close, it looks as if he's her boyfriend, so I decide to forge ahead. "It's a long story which doesn't make much sense. It involves some confidential medical records. Did you recently have a medical test done in McMinnville?"

Mallory sways a little on her feet and sits back down on the wooden park bench. She looks back and forth between Andre and me and nods. "Umm … yeah, I had a mammogram a few weeks ago."

"You good here, Mal?" Andre asks. "I don't need to hear about your ta-tas. If this guy passes muster, I'll go chill with Philip. He's leaving town tomorrow to start another job."

Mallory waves him off. "I'm fine. Go!"

Andre kisses her cheek and hugs her goodbye. "Be gentle with this guy — he seems nice."

Chapter Six

Mallory

I SNEAK A PEEK over Andre's shoulder as he gives me a hug. This time, it's Rocco who is watching our interaction with an amused expression. After Andre jogs off to meet Philip, Rocco comments, "Your boyfriend seems concerned about my well-being. Is there something I should know?"

I bite back a snort of laughter. "Andre is not my boyfriend. Never has been. He's my assistant. He keeps my business life running smoothly. Truth be told, he keeps my personal life on track too — but that's not officially his job, he just does it because he's awesome."

Rocco smiles, and it changes him from a merely interesting looking guy to devastatingly handsome. "Oh, I get it. He's here to play the big brother role, right? Smart."

I grin. "For someone who is totally not related to me, you'd be surprised how often he steps into those shoes." I stop and take a deep breath. "Okay, I think I've stalled enough. Tell me how in the world you could possibly know I had a mammogram."

Rocco's expression grows instantly serious as he shrugs off a backpack he has slung over his shoulder. He pulls out a large manila envelope and hands over an accordion file.

"A few weeks ago, I got this in the mail, out of the blue. I thought it was from HR. I'm a paramedic and sometimes I pick up extra hours by working medical transport for the hospital. I recently completed enough hours to qualify for class bump. I thought they were notifying me I got a pay raise. I was startled when it turned out to be your mammogram results. So, I read the report to see if I could figure out why I received the information."

I hold up my hand to stop him from talking. My brain is trying to catch up with his words. I am frantically scanning the file he gave me to try to make sense of it all. When I agreed to have this mammogram to settle Edna's nerves, I didn't even realize they were actually taking real pictures. I thought they simply went through the motions. I'm not even thirty! I'm decades away from actually needing a mammogram. As far as I know, I don't have any family history of breast cancer. Then again when you're adopted, your family history is whatever your social worker says it is. It may or may not be true.

I look up at Rocco as I fight to maintain my composure. "I majored in English. I know what this says. Bear with me as I ask a really dumb question." I pause to angrily wipe away tears. "Does this say what I think it says? Does this stupid piece of paper say I am dying of cancer?"

I jump when Rocco reaches out and takes both of my hands between his and forcefully answers, "No!" He squeezes my hands for emphasis before he continues.

"That piece of paper says a lot of things — many of them are untrue. It doesn't say you are going to die. Okay? It's not over." He focuses on my expression with laser intensity as if he can will this all to go away.

"Are you saying I might not have cancer? This all might be one huge mistake?"

He rolls his shoulder. "I suppose anything is possible. However, it's unlikely since you actually had a mammogram recently."

I pause to reread the report again. "This is crazy! It says we're married. I've never laid eyes on you before today. Why would they have your name on my medical records?"

"I don't know. Remember when I told you some of the report is fiction? There are a lot of things I don't understand — starting with why you had a mammogram at your age. Did your doctor think you were at some special risk?"

I shake my head in frustration. "No! It's one of those stories that's too weird to be believed."

Rocco leans back against the park bench. "It's my day off. I'm in no hurry —"

I smirk. "Well, it's not as if I've got any secrets from you at this point anyway. My parents live on the East Coast where my dad's a dentist. He was hoping I would go to dental school and take over his practice, so he and Mom could retire and live somewhere exotic like Paris. Unfortunately, all the stories he told me growing up didn't inspire me to be a dentist — they just grossed me out. My favorite English teacher in high school used to be a newspaper reporter, so the bug hit early. My parents were profoundly disappointed that I didn't want to carry on the family legacy. They practically disowned me over my decision, so I moved about as far away from Maine as I possibly could."

"I'm sorry. That sounds awful. My mom gets distressed if I don't bring laundry over every week for her to do."

I burst out laughing. "Seriously? How old are you? Are you telling me you don't know how to do your own laundry?"

Rocco blushes bright red. "I didn't say I didn't know how to do my own laundry. I just have to talk my mom into allowing me to do it. The whole situation is awkward. I don't want to hurt her feelings but she doesn't want to let me grow up. She doesn't seem to understand that I'm twenty-six and my brother Remy is thirty-one."

"I shouldn't tease you. I am in a similar quandary. It's actually the reason why I've undergone several random medical tests recently," I confess with the look of chagrin.

Rocco raises an eyebrow. "Okay, I know there must be a story there somewhere."

"There is. I hope you weren't kidding about not being in a hurry. This is a little convoluted. After I graduated from college, I got a great job. You know, the kind career offices like to tout as their finest success stories? I was chosen from hundreds of applicants. I really liked my job too —"

"Why do I have this overwhelming hunch there is a huge but at the end of that sentence?"

I sigh as I wrap my coat tighter around myself. "It was all going phenomenally well until the boss threatened to hire his niece for my position instead of me."

Rocco frowns. "Just like that?"

"Oh, he gave me a chance to save my job. All I had to do was agree to sleep with him."

"What a disgusting cad! Couldn't you file charges or something? That has to be illegal!"

"It is — but remember I was fresh out of college. I was the new kid on the block and he was senior management. It was his word against mine. He made sure there were no witnesses."

"Of course he did. That's what jerks like him do. I feel like I need to apologize for my entire gender."

I wince. "I hate to tell you this. The story gets even worse. So, since I lost my plum, high-paying job I had to move in with a couple of good friends from college. At first it worked out okay. I did some tutoring and test proctoring. I even sold makeup at the mall. It wasn't glamorous, but I was making ends meet."

"Still, it had to be discouraging to graduate from college and end up working in jobs like that."

"It was. But I was just buying time until the right job came along. My grades in college were stellar, so I was sure I could land another position soon."

"What happened?"

"One of my roommates decided to become obsessed with the other one. Even though we had all been just friends for years, JR suddenly decided Juliette wasn't free to date. When she tried to go out, he attempted to kill her."

"You wouldn't believe how many domestic violence calls we respond to. It's horrifying."

"After testifying at his trial, nothing shocks me

anymore. The whole experience shaped my career. I used to think I might be interested in covering politics. In a way, I guess I still do. But now I focus on how political decisions impact crime."

"That's all very interesting. But it doesn't explain your random medical tests," Rocco says with a puzzled look.

"I told you it was convoluted," I explain. "After the trial, Juliette couldn't stand to live in the house where she was attacked. My grandma had recently passed away and gave me a small inheritance and I used the money to purchase the house from Juliette's parents. They were just happy to get it out of their hands, so they let me have it for dirt cheap. I remodeled the whole thing."

"It's a terrible way to get a house, but a nice way to turn around a bad situation." He seems to struggle to find the right words to say.

"Before the trial, the police department warned my elderly neighbor, Edna, that she should be on the lookout for unusual activity. She took it upon herself to become an amateur sleuth. She considered it her responsibility to watch out for me. Of course, I didn't learn about this until years after the fact. Edna made up reasons to check up on me. She brought over meals and fresh food from her garden. Edna would bring over her dog for me to visit in case I was lonely. Soon, she started stopping by my place a couple times a day just for coffee. When she found out my parents live clear across the United States, she made me one of her honorary grandchildren. She buys me gifts for every holiday — not just Christmas but like Arbor Day."

"How cool is that? I bet she makes amazing cookies, doesn't she?"

"Oh, you have no idea! At Christmas time, I eat so many sugar cookies I practically need a crane to get me back over to my house. So, you can see why I feel like I owe Edna the world."

Rocco nods sympathetically. "Yeah, I get it."

"It started out small. First, Edna needed new shoes, and she wanted me to take her shopping. Nothing wrong with that, right? That's all pretty normal. Then, she had to go in for some sort of x-ray where she had to drink barium. She was afraid it would make her throw up. She wanted me to talk to her in the waiting room to keep her calm. I figured it was the nice thing to do. So, I went with her. I've never seen anyone shake so bad over having to drink a small cup of fluid. I thought she would pass out."

"Wow! I wonder if she had a previous bad experience?"

"The next time she asked me to go on a strange outing; she told me she was scared to go to the eye doctor because they were planning to dilate her eyes. She has glaucoma and she needs it tested routinely. All of a sudden, she wanted me to have an eye exam because her doctor was retiring. She wanted me to check out the new doctor to see if he was okay. Reluctantly, I agreed because she was so afraid of her last medical procedure. I guess it's a good thing I went. My contact lens needed an adjustment because it was putting pressure on my cornea."

"Sounds like it was a good call."

"I thought the eye doctor would be the end of it, but then she wanted me to get a mammogram with her. She steadfastly refused to get one unless I went with her. At her age, I knew it was an important test, so I went for what I thought was an inconsequential test. Edna was so nervous, and it seemed like such a small thing to make her happy — I wasn't even sure they did a full mammogram. When I never got results, I thought maybe the whole thing was just an elaborate charade."

Rocco runs his hand through his hair. He reaches for the file as he asks, "May I?"

Confused, I hand it back to him. He scoots closer to me and pulls a pen from the inside pocket of his jacket. He pulls what looks like an x-ray film out of the file. He holds it up to the sunlight. "I know you think this was all some big screw up on the part of the hospital, but this strange comedy of errors might just save your life." Rocco points to what looks like a white shadow on my left breast. "Like I said, I'm not really a doctor, but I scored quite well on all my anatomy and physiology stuff in my paramedic course work. If money was no object, I probably would've gone to medical school. The way the body works, or in this case, doesn't work — fascinates me. I suspect this area is what caused the radiologist to have concern in your case. He gave you a BI-RADS score of five. It means the radiologist is ninety-five percent sure you've got an issue which requires further study."

"Let's be honest, all that is just a polite way to say I've got cancer, right?"

"Nothing is definitive quite yet. It could simply be an anomaly on your mammogram — but, you need to have a look at it, for sure."

"How is this even happening to me? I wasn't supposed to have a mammogram for a couple decades. I have too much to do to have cancer. I can't die! I'm on the verge of proving a young man has been incarcerated for a crime he didn't commit. Why does this have to happen right now?"

"My best friend died from leukemia when I was nine. There is never a good time to get cancer and no matter how hard you try, you can't make sense of it. You might as well not waste your energy trying."

A million thoughts race around in my brain. "I love my job, Rocco, but *Word Soup PNW* is just a little upstart paper. Our health insurance benefits are almost nonexistent. What am I going to do? Passion for my job doesn't cover medical bills!"

I tremble as panic sets in. A tear slides down my cheek and Rocco reaches up and wipes it away with the pad of his thumb.

"I don't know all the answers. But, one of my good friends is a doctor. Jaxson's specialty is orthopedics, but he can steer us in the right direction. If he doesn't know the right answer, he can find us someone who does."

I pull away and look at Rocco incredulously. "We? I know the paperwork says we're married, but the truth is we are still strangers and you're not responsible for me. You can walk away and pretend we never met."

Rocco shakes his head. "I suppose I could, but unless you want me to — I'd rather not."

"Why on earth would you want to stick around? Whatever happens, it won't be fun."

"Well, I'm not a huge believer in random coincidence. I figure there was a reason I was plopped into the middle of your life, so I might as well stick around and see why I was invited to the party. Besides, you probably could use an extra friend or two."

Rocco's words bring me up short. "That's the strangest thing I've ever heard. I need to think about it for a while. I have so much to consider. My whole life has been turned upside down."

Rocco reaches out, grasps my hands and gives them a squeeze. "I understand. You know how to get hold of me. If it goes to voice mail, I'm not ignoring you — it just means I'm on shift. I'll get back to you as soon as I can."

------●------

Andre lays his chopsticks down on the edge of his plate and leans back in his chair. "Mal, I get why you're freaked out about the cancer thing. Anybody in their right mind would be." He leans forward and takes a sip of his ice water. "But, you have to run this whole thing about Rocco by me again — because from the cheap seats, it looks like the dude has been nothing but perfect. If I were in your shoes, I'm not so sure I'd be so quick to kick him to the curb."

I stick my tongue out at Andre. "Oh shut up! You're only saying that because you think he's cute. What would Philip say?"

"My amazing fiancé would compliment me on my good taste. He thought Rocco was scorching hot too. You didn't notice him taking a few candid shots the other night? Philip is almost finished with the portrait he's been working on. He was searching around for his next subject. Your knight in shining armor might perfectly fit the bill."

I scoff. "Rocco is hardly my knight in shining armor. If anything, he's more like my own personal Grim Reaper."

"I don't know. I'm starting to change my opinion about the guy — and not simply because he's adorable. He worked awfully hard to reach you. I didn't make it easy to get to you and he wasn't dissuaded. If he didn't care about you, he could've thrown the file in the trash and not thought another thing about it. So, in my book he gets bonus points for going above and beyond the call of duty to be a better-than-average citizen."

I sigh. "But why? Why would someone like him do something like that for me?"

Andre shrugs. "As hard as it may be to believe — especially in our line of work — maybe he is just that nice."

"What do you think of his theory that our paths crossed because we were destined to meet or something?"

"It's either that or a straight up miracle. There's no other plausible explanation for all of this."

I stare long and hard at Andre. "Pardon my skepticism, but I find it hard to believe anything to do with cancer could be considered a miracle."

"I understand. I also know you've been telling me you wish you had more friends in Oregon. This guy is offering you the chance to make more connections here, what could it hurt to reach out? You just have to fight your natural shyness and go out on a limb. I think you should. I bet he's one of the good guys."

"The question is … will I even be here long enough to find out for certain?"

"That may be a whole different kind of fight. But, I have a feeling Rocco Pierce would happily stand by your side if you invite him to be there."

CHAPTER SEVEN

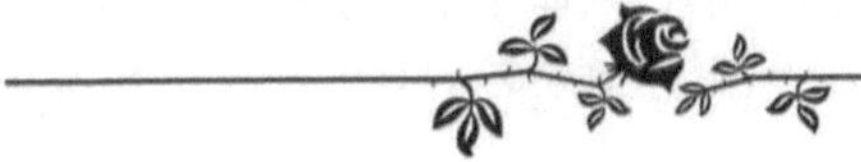

ROCCO

I SCOOP A BOX off of my parents' porch on the way through the door. "UPS driver was here early," I comment as I place the box in front of my dad before I grab a cup of coffee. When my dad sees the return address, he grins. "Oh, great! Your mother's Christmas present came. Maybe you should hide this at your apartment. She always snoops out my best hiding places." Finally, my dad looks up at me. "Geez! You look awful. Long night?"

I nod. "We had back-to-back fatals. First, there were a bunch of kids drag racing while drunk. One of them flipped the car and damn-near decapitated themselves. There was nothing I could do there. They were dead before we ever pulled up. Blood-alcohol count was twice the legal limit."

"Some people never learn," my dad mutters. "Booze and cars never mix."

"I no sooner cleared that scene when I was called out again. I'm not even sure why PD called us. Maybe they thought we could do some good. We tried resuscitation, but it was far too late. A mom and her eighteen-month-old daughter died of carbon monoxide poisoning. It appears as if she was trying to heat the house with a gas oven. I'm not sure if it was a malfunction or what, but PD found them with the oven door open and all bundled up. Raylene and I couldn't save them."

"Oh son, I'm so sorry. Are the police investigating what killed those poor people?" my dad asks with a look of sympathy.

"I honestly don't know, Dad. It seemed pretty straightforward on scene."

"That's a real shame. Nobody should have to die simply to stay warm."

"I agree." I take a long sip of coffee and try to mentally shake off my shift.

"Want some breakfast? I'm about ready to fry up some eggs and bacon."

"Sure. I just stopped by to pick up my laundry."

My phone beeps and I check my messages. I can't hide my smile from my dad. "Good news?" he asks as he walks toward the refrigerator.

"The best I've had in a while. It seems I've just picked up a late lunch date with Mallory."

"Mallory? Is she the gal your mom was telling me about with cancer?"

"Well, I don't know for sure she has cancer, but she probably does." I choose my words carefully.

"Seems to me that would be something a person would know, wouldn't they?" my dad asks with a puzzled expression.

"Probably in a normal situation, but nothing about

this has been normal. It's complicated."

"Are you sure you want to get involved? Doesn't your job have enough drama?"

"I already am involved. Strangely enough, I'm in no hurry to get uninvolved. I feel drawn to Mallory — even before I met her I felt compelled to find her. Now that I have connected with her, I can't get her off of my mind."

My dad examines me closely from head to toe. "I know you didn't ask my opinion, but if you want to catch this young lady's attention, you better go home and get some rest, get cleaned up and go visit yourself a barber. You are looking a little rough around the edges."

"Haven't you heard? Women find the rugged look sexy these days," I comment as I rub my fingers over my admittedly long stubble.

"There's rugged and then there's Sasquatch's cousin. I think you crossed that line a few days back, son."

"Good point. I'll stop by and see Stan before lunch."

"Do you need your mother to give you a refresher on table manners?"

"No, I think I've got it. I'm not completely uncivilized."

"Your mother is very concerned about how much fast food you eat. She sees the receipts in your pockets when she does your laundry. Why is your mother doing your laundry, by the way?"

"Have you ever tried to talk her out of something?" I counter with a laugh.

My dad shakes his head in resignation. "Good point. I'll see you next week when you drop your next load off. You can tell me how your date went then."

Mallory erupts in a fit of giggles as my shot bounces so wide it goes into the gravel beside the course. "Nothing personal Rocco, but I hope your aim is better when you handle needles."

"Inserting IVs is a completely different skill set than playing miniature golf. Besides, I'm a tad sleep deprived."

Mallory looks dismayed as she covers her mouth. "Why didn't you say something? I just burst into your life and demanded an audience like I'm royalty. I didn't even think about the fact you might have worked graveyard."

I reach up and tuck her hair behind her ear. "Mallory, don't worry about it. I am exactly where I want to be." Out of the corner of my eye, I see our waitress walk toward our table on the covered patio. "Looks like our food has arrived. Shall we?" I offer to take her golf club.

She hands it to me and smiles. "Sure. I'm starving."

As we're walking toward our table, a woman abruptly scoots her chair back into the pathway. I place my hand on the small of Mallory's back and guide her around the intrusion. When we reach the table, I pull out the chair for her and help her out of her jacket.

After I sit down and place my napkin on my lap, she studies me with open curiosity. "I have been on some interesting dates lately. Rarely does anyone impress me so quickly. You're off to a good start."

"That's good to hear. I had to make up for my less than heroic performance at mini-golf."

Mallory takes a couple bites of her salad. "This is amazing. Thanks for not hassling me for ordering salad on a date. I just like salad for lunch. It's been a long time since I've had a good Caesar salad. Listen to me babble."

I squeeze her hand in what I hope is a reassuring gesture. "It looks good. Perhaps I'll order it next time we come here."

"Maybe I'm not ready for this conversation after all. I'm sorry for bothering you when you should be sleeping. Thank you for lunch though. It's just the break from reality I need right now." She turns away and tries to hide her face as she wipes away tears with the back of her hand.

I hand her a napkin. "It sounds like you could use a shoulder to lean on. My offer of friendship still stands."

Mallory sets down her fork and turns toward me with an intense, somber expression. "You may be sorry you ever opened that stupid letter —" she lets her speech trail off.

"I don't see it that way at all. I don't know what happened, but the hospital didn't have you in their computerized systems. So, if I hadn't gotten your record, you may never have received your results. It was a good thing bits and bytes got scrambled in cyberspace."

Mallory sighs. "Results. I wish I had actual results. The only thing I have is someone's guess that there might be a problem. I don't even know what to do with that. I feel so frustrated. I'm stuck. I don't know where to go from here."

"I hope you don't mind. I talked to my friend, Dr. Jaxson Shepherd. His mom had breast cancer awhile back. She's fine now. Come to think of it, his mother-in-law had lung cancer a few years ago too."

"Did she survive?" Mallory asks anxiously.

"Yes, Gwendolyn is more than five years cancer free.

Her oncologist gave me the number of someone she recommends for the treatment of breast cancer."

"Wow! You didn't have to do any of that stuff. You barely know me," Mallory stammers.

"I promised you I wouldn't just dump bad news in your lap and then split."

"I guess not. So, do I start with the specialist?"

"Jax says you should have an ultrasound and another mammogram done to confirm the test results were valid and that the mammogram results are actually yours."

"Easy for him to say. He's a doctor with medical insurance out the wazoo. He can have as many medical tests as he wants."

"At least for right now, I wouldn't worry about it. The records department has a lot of explaining to do. The whole radiology department is bending over backwards to make sure you are a happy customer. Currently, making you happy means keeping your 'husband' calm."

Mallory's mouth gapes open. "You didn't!"

I shrug. "Not in so many words. When I was trying to locate you, they made a copy of the information they sent me. Apparently, a staff member input it into the computer verbatim. The person I spoke to at the front desk who knows I'm not your husband, doesn't appear to work in the records department anymore. I can't help it if the new staff made assumptions."

Mallory shuts her eyes and shakes her head in disbelief. "Why do I have this sinking feeling this might come back to haunt me later? It's funny, journalists have a reputation for being sneaky — but even I wouldn't have thought of trying that. Are you sure they won't charge me for the tests?"

I nod. I queue up a voicemail from the hospital. "Hi, this is April Williamson from Guest Relations. I'm just following up regarding a possible miscommunication your wife had between our Records Department and Radiology. We, of course, would be happy to provide any follow-up imaging your wife needs to set her mind at ease. We regret any inconvenience this incident has caused. We'd like to contact your wife, but our records seem to be somewhat incomplete. Please pass this message on to her at your earliest opportunity."

Just like it did the first time I heard it, the cavalier attitude of the administration still shocks me and makes me instantly furious. I watch Mallory carefully as she absorbs the words.

Mallory grows quiet as she chews on the edge of her fingernail. She looks up at me with a horrified expression. "'Inconvenience'? Is that what we're calling the terrifying upheaval my life has undergone in the last couple of weeks?"

She hiccups and lets out a quiet sob before she takes a sip of water. "Do you know that I went to a funeral home and looked at options for coffins, just so my parents wouldn't have to? That's more than just a little inconvenient."

"I wish you would have said something. That's not something you should have to do alone — or at all just yet. You don't even know for certain if you have breast cancer or how bad it is. I think you should start at the beginning and get further testing."

"Intellectually, I know. I'm a reporter, for Pete's sake. I know how to gather facts and confirm a hypothesis. I know how important it is to get information from multiple sources. Yet, I can't seem to bring myself to pick up the phone to make an appointment. I don't know what's wrong with me."

I reach out and grasp Mallory's hands and place them between my own. They are freezing, even though we are sitting in front of the fireplace and it is a relatively warm fall day. "Don't you think you are being a tad hard on yourself? This isn't about some story objective. This is your life. I blindsided you with news you never expected to hear. Your response is perfectly logical given the circumstances."

Mallory shakes her head. "No, it's not! You're a health care professional. You know I need to get treatment for whatever this is. Otherwise you would not have worked so hard to make sure I got the results of my test, right?"

I've never been a very good poker player. So, I nod slowly. "Early detection gives you the best odds. But, if you need a few days to wrap your mind around all of this, that's understandable."

"That's what scares me. I don't know how much time I have. I had a professor in college who came to class on a Monday and told us he found out he had pancreatic cancer. Three weeks later, he was dead."

"Mallory, you can't think that way. First, pancreatic cancer and breast cancer are very different things. Second, you are young and healthy. We are not even sure what the radiologist saw on your mammogram. It may still turn out to be nothing. You won't know that for sure until you have more testing."

"At the risk of sounding like my neighbor, Edna, I'm not sure I'm strong enough to face this on my own. Still, I'm reluctant to involve my parents at this point in case it turns out to be nothing."

"Lucky for you, you happen to have a spare husband lying around with more vacation hours socked away than he knows what to do with."

"Very funny. In case no one bothered to inform you, that was just a paperwork glitch. You are not actually my husband. You don't have to hold my hand through all of this. I've been doing some Internet research. This process can get grizzly — even the initial diagnosis stage can involve needles and scalpels."

"I knew what I was signing up for the minute I saw the report. It's okay. I see grizzly every day. I can handle it. It's up to you whether you want to tell them I am your real husband or just your friend. Either way, I am here for you as long as you want me to be."

Mallory is silent for a few moments as she studies me as I eat. "Are you really this nice? What's wrong with you? I mean why aren't you married for real?"

I pause as I take a drink of my coffee. "That's a good question. I think about it every time one of my buddies gets married. I guess I don't have any great answers other than I work crazy hours and hang out a lot with my parents and my friends who are married. They've all tried to match me up with their single friends. But I just haven't found anybody who I had things in common with and who understood my dedication to my job. In a way, I've become the weird cat guy who likes to come home and read books and hang out with my cat when I'm not working. I've become a sad stereotype before I even hit thirty."

Mallory giggles. "Welcome to the club. Remember when we were teenagers and we thought being a grown-up was so glamorous?"

I smirk. "Tell me about it! The other day I was alone in my apartment with my cat, Chevy, and I said something out loud that was such a ringer for something my dad would say I had to look around to see if he was in the room with me."

"So, where do we go from here?"

I pull my wallet out of my back pocket and fish a card out of it. "Here is Dr. Callie Stephenson's card. She is a surgeon who specializes in breast cancer. Jax says her office will want an ultrasound first. Her medical assistant is Dixie. She can help you schedule any testing you need. Just let me know what you have set up, and I'll be there."

"So that's it?" Mallory responds with a sigh. "My life has been reduced to a series of lies? We are going to pretend to be a happily married couple going about our business living life like everything's hunky-dory until the other shoe officially drops and the final verdict is in?"

I smile at her sarcastic assessment of the situation. She would fit in well as a paramedic. Sometimes we use dark humor to cope with emotionally charged situations as well. "I might have put it a little differently, but that about sums it up. I can arrange for you to have dinner with my parents and play bingo at church game night if you want to stretch the scenario out even further," I suggest with my tongue firmly in my cheek.

Mallory looks at me blankly for a moment and then laughs out loud. "Heck, we might as well invite Edna too. Why keep our delusion to ourselves? We should have a huge block party, right? This whole thing is patently ludicrous. If anyone knew what we were planning, they would come after us with straitjackets. This is insane! You can't pretend to be my husband simply because some paperwork glitch somewhere says you are."

I shrug. "Why not? I know of some real-life marriages being held together by far less."

"Because it's a lie and lying is wrong!" Mallory insists.

"Okay, so we don't lie. We'll introduce me by my name. If they make assumptions based on the information they have on file, we'll let it stand. If they ask us questions about our relationship, I'll say I'm there to support you as your friend. Deal?"

Mallory nods slowly. "Sounds like a good compromise to me. I don't think I can handle this alone. I'm grateful you decided to step up."

Mallory grips my hand tightly as we drive for the hospital. "Are you sure it's such a great idea for us to come back here? They made a big mess of things the first time."

I flip on my blinker to change lanes. "I had the same concern, so I asked Dixie about it specifically. Although she doesn't know what to make of your specific situation, she said it was a good idea to have your follow-up exams done in same facility so the radiologists can compare results. I have a feeling they don't want to mess with Sergeant Dixie. She was a triage medic in Operation Desert Shield. She'll make sure they fly right. "

"What did you do? A whole background check?"

"No, nothing that complicated. Dr. Stephenson's office happens to be in the same professional complex as Dr. Shepherd's. I popped over there when I returned

Jaxson's phone charger. Dixie had a picture behind her desk. I had seen many pictures like that growing up since my dad served in Desert Storm. It was a natural topic of conversation."

"I know what you mean. Dixie is so easy to talk to. For the first time since I found out about this, she made it all seem manageable. Still, I'm not sure I won't freak out in the middle of the exam and run out of the room screaming."

"How can I help you the most?" I gently squeeze her hand. "I'll do anything you need me to do."

"I don't know! We haven't even been on a date. You just met me a couple of weeks ago. It'll be super weird if you're in there while they're examining every square inch of my breasts, wouldn't it?"

"Only if you think it's weird."

"Rocco, be serious!"

"I am being serious. Listen, I'm a paramedic. You have no idea the weirdness I see in my job. This doesn't even hit the Richter scale. I once went on a call where some guy put a goldfish in his rectum. Now, that was weird."

"Seriously? How drunk was he?"

"Sadly, he was stone cold sober. He had watched some porn flick and gotten an idea that it might be sexy."

Mallory shudders. "I don't suppose he found the experience as satisfying as he hoped?"

I shake my head. "Trips to the ER rarely are. Besides, as far as the technician knows, I'm already your husband. Nobody would think twice about me being there."

"But I would know you're not my husband," Mallory

argues as she lets out an exasperated breath. "That's what makes it weird. We've never even kissed and you'll be seeing me half naked."

I pull my car into the parking spot and take my phone out of my glove box. I glance at the time and wink at Mallory. "We're plenty early. We could take care of that little issue."

Her eyes widen. "What little issue?" she asks with trepidation.

"If you're worried that we haven't kissed, I'm happy to take care of that."

Mallory lets loose with a surprised gust of laughter. "That's the worst come-on line I've ever heard. Trust me, my bar isn't very high. I work with a bunch of twenty-somethings who don't get out much."

I point at myself in a gesture of feigned innocence. "Who, me? It wasn't my idea — you're the one who brought it up."

Mallory bites her bottom lip. "Oh right. I did. Good point. If you're planning to pretend to be my husband, we probably should act like we're more than perfect strangers. Maybe a kiss or two wouldn't be such a bad idea," she mumbles, half under her breath.

I chuckle when I see Mallory's pensive expression. "You don't have to make it seem like it's a fate worse than eating overcooked broccoli or something. The women down at the firehouse say I kiss pretty well." I take off my seatbelt and walk around the car to help Mallory out of the car.

As she takes my hand to stand up she asks, "I thought guys weren't supposed to brag about that kind of stuff — and how would they know?"

"I swear, it was for good cause. We were raising money for the Muscular Dystrophy Association. The firefighters and the paramedics got a little competitive when it came to the kissing booth. I think they got a little overconfident because their uniforms are sexier than ours, but in a surprise upset, we were voted the 'hottest kissers'."

Mallory turns around and walks backwards as she faces me. "Funny thing about me … It's annoying … really. It drives all my friends nuts — but, I don't ever take anyone's word at face value. I always have to confirm things independently."

I raise an eyebrow. "Oh, is that so?"

"Definitely." Mallory stops so abruptly in front of me I have to put my arms around her to prevent us both from falling down.

I can't help but notice how comfortably she fits in my arms as if she was always meant to be there. For a moment I tuck her under my chin. "I know a charming spot not far away. Would you like to take a walk?"

I feel her nod against my chin.

We walk in silence through a few side streets and alleys.

As I steer Mallory around a deep pothole in the bleak alley we are traversing, she stops and glances up with a worried expression. "I know you're supposed to be here to make me feel more comfortable today. I'm not exactly feeling safe here."

"Give me a couple minutes and your view will change dramatically, I promise."

"Rocco, I'm not kidding. I am petrified. I don't even want to be here today. I don't want to think about all the things that could go wrong today. This is not a good day to play some weird practical joke on me."

The scent of roses fills the air as I stop in front of a large white wooden gate. I unlock the intricate wrought iron latch and place my hand in the small of Mallory's back as I escort her through the opening. "Are you sure we're supposed to be —" Her speech trails off as she glances around the lush rose garden with its eclectic collection of birdbaths.

"I'm positive," I respond as I walk her over to the Adirondack chairs in the gazebo next to the fire pit. "I often come out here when I need to get my mind off a stressful day."

"I can see why — but you can't go barging into a stranger's yard," she warns.

I run my hand down the carved pillar of the gazebo. "My dad and I built this for my mom for Mother's Day. I've always wanted to show it to someone special."

Mallory swallows hard. "You brought me to meet your parents on one of the most stressful days of my life? Do you know they told me not to wear deodorant? Tell me you did not do this to me! I'm not ready to meet anybody. How do we even explain what's going on between us? I don't even know what's going on between us."

I reach out and touch Mallory's face with my hands. "Relax. My parents are not here. Today they are making a Costco run. They are always gone for hours when they run to town. My dad is planning to take my mom out to dinner tonight. I would not spring my parents on you without plenty of advance warning."

"Why? What's wrong with them?" Mallory asks as

she sinks down and sits on the edge of the Adirondack chair.

I sit down beside her and laugh at her blunt question. "Nothing — as long as you're prepared to play twenty questions on steroids — or have my mom assume we're going to get married tomorrow. My mom used to be a hairdresser. She can talk to anybody about anything. My dad used to be a supply clerk in the military. When he came back, he sold office equipment to businesses all up and down the valley. When his company started hitting tough times, he took an option for early retirement. He is a little more reserved than my mom, but he has the gift of gab too. Between the two of them, it's a little difficult to have many secrets."

Mallory sags against me a little. "Does that mean they know what's going on between us?"

"They have a rough idea. At first, I was concerned that the mammogram results were somehow tied to my mom. I had to explain why I was asking about her most recent test."

Mallory chokes back a laugh. "I bet that was a conversation you weren't expecting to have with your mom."

"She was a tad surprised at my question. Then again, to quote her, 'You've always been a weird child.'"

"Surprisingly, despite the weirdness of the situation, you've been one of the nicest guys I've ever met."

"I hope that means you won't mind if I do this," I murmur as I lean close and brush a light kiss across her lips.

Mallory pulls away and looks up at me with a bemused expression. "That wasn't as weird as I expected it to be."

"Thank you — I think."

"No, it was totally a compliment. You wouldn't believe how awkward first kisses can be. Maybe we should try it again just to make sure it wasn't a fluke." After a moment she adds, "Let's stand up. Sometimes my lack of height can be a challenge."

I stand up and reach my hand out to help her up. "That's not a problem. I thrive on challenges."

I thread my fingers through her shiny black hair and tilt her face up toward mine as I lean down and kiss her a little more thoroughly. "I could get used to that. I see no problems with your height. But, if your neck gets sore, I could always pick you up like this and kiss you some more." I scoop her up and hold her close as I kiss her one more time. I'm totally lost in the sensation of her soft lips against mine when I hear an odd beeping.

"Oh, shoot! Of all the times for reality to intrude into my life. I had almost forgotten why we're here. We've got ten minutes to get to my appointment. I guess we won't have to pretend we've got good chemistry between the two of us. Maybe our chemistry is too good for a married couple," she jokes as she straightens her clothes after I set her back down on the ground.

"I don't know. We could always claim we're newlyweds. One of the guys at the fire station recently got married and when his new wife comes to visit the two of them are all over each other. It's plausible."

"I don't even know what to think. On one hand, I wish I would never have gone near a mammogram machine or heard of breast cancer. Yet, if this had never happened, I would've never met you —"

"I know what you mean. I feel the same way when I think about the letter. It's amazing to think how much it's changed both of our lives already. Just know I'm here for you whatever happens."

"I know. I've never been so scared and so hopeful at the same time."

CHAPTER EIGHT

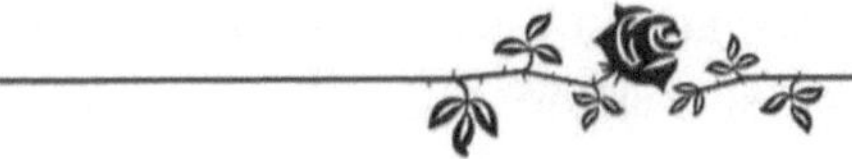

MALLORY

I drum my fingers against my kitchen counter as I try to ignore the blueberry muffins Edna left for me. I feel terrible. I know she knows something is wrong. But I don't know what to tell her. If I spill the whole story, I'm sure she'll feel guilty because she is the one who persuaded me to get a mammogram. I don't even have any news yet and it's driving me crazy.

Desperate, I pull my phone out of my pocket and call Rocco. "Please tell me I haven't interrupted you in the middle of a life and death call," I blurt when he sounds distracted.

"No, that's not it at all. I'm simply trying to keep my parents' boxer, Sugar Ray, from eating the charcoal briquettes that are falling out of the bag. He thinks he's helping my dad set up the barbecue. He is a sweet dog, but he's not so bright."

"Sounds like fun! I love dogs. I'm planning to get one of my own soon."

"Do you want to come over? My mom has been

marinating chicken for the grill. It'll be delicious."

"I probably shouldn't. I would be terrible company — I am a nervous wreck waiting for the results. I don't understand what's taking them so long to read a simple ultrasound. It must be catastrophic news."

"Try not to read too much into it. You never know how many emergencies have come in or who got bumped ahead of you. You should join us. It'll be a great diversion."

I sigh. "I might as well. It's not like I'm getting anything done here. I should be reading materials for work — but I can't concentrate on anything."

"Sounds like you need a mental health break. Do you like music? A group of my friends are getting together to go to a concert tonight. It's a little country, a little jazz, a little folk music. It's awesome."

I choke on my Sprite and almost drop my phone. "Rocco, throwing on some cutoffs and a tank top so I can have a barbecue with your parents is one thing. Getting ready to go out for a concert with your friends when they've never met me is a whole other level of preparation. How would we explain whatever is going on between us?"

"I know you've probably been told this before, but my friends are totally chill. Don't worry about explaining our relationship to them. In fact a few of them even know the basics because they helped me track you down."

I groan into the phone. "Like that won't be all kinds of awkward. I don't think you understand how high the stakes are when women make friends. First impressions are everything. Women plan for weeks before they go to a concert. Wardrobe choice is key."

"I doubt if it's too important in this venue. Think a couple of notches above a coffee shop."

"If you're sure, I'd love to come. Would your mom mind if I bring some blueberry muffins?"

"She'd love it, but my dad would love you even more. Blueberry muffins are one of his favorites. Mom was planning dinner around three since the concert starts at six. I'm sure my dad will appreciate the extra goodies."

"I will pack a few extra just for him. See you later."

<hr>

"You are a lucky woman Mrs. Pierce," I comment as Rocco brings me a tall glass of ice-cold strawberry lemonade and Mr. Pierce places a bowl of fresh, plump berries between us. She hands me a small paper plate and pushes a sugar bowl in my direction.

She smiles as her eyes follow her husband until he leaves our line of sight. "You are right. I am incredibly blessed," she comments as she turns back toward me. "I don't know about you, but I like my fruit with a little powdered sugar on the top. Call me Veronica, or Ronnie. Rocco's father is Richard, but the only person to call him that is his father. Everyone else calls him Rick."

"It's a pleasure to meet you, Veronica. You have such a beautiful rose garden. I especially love your cherry trees."

"I was so surprised to receive the pictures of you and Rocco in my flower garden. For such a sweet, outgoing guy, Rocco is quite camera shy. I never get him to smile for photographs — but you got some lovely pictures of him. I can't tell you how much I appreciate it. How did you pull it off?"

I look across the lawn at Rocco who is playing Frisbee with Sugar Ray. I grin at the comical expression on the boxer's face as the toy dangles from his mouth.

"To be honest, I only got those great pictures because your son was being incredibly sweet to me on one of the toughest days I've had in a while. I had to have some testing done at the hospital, and Rocco volunteered to go with me to keep me calm."

Veronica nods. "Yes, he told me a bit about the paperwork problems."

I grimace. "It's awful, isn't it? But the funny thing is, your son isn't treating it like it's devastating news. That's how we got the great pictures. After my test, I was feeling completely stressed out. So, he brought me back to your beautiful garden for an impromptu yoga session and a bit of positive thinking meditation. So, he let me take pictures of him — hundreds and hundreds of pictures. Some of them were serious, others were goofy. Many were sweet and touching. It's almost as if he's actually the husband the hospital thinks he is."

"Would that be so terrible?" Veronica presses. "Rocco needs someone in his life. He carries so many burdens on those wide shoulders of his. He needs a soulmate to share his life with."

"I'm sorry. I like your son — a lot. More than I ever dreamed I could. But, I don't think I'm soulmate material right now. There's a good chance I might not live long enough to see my thirtieth birthday."

"Oh dear, is that what the tests said? Rocco didn't mention anything to me about the results." Veronica answers as tears spring to her eyes.

"Oh, don't cry, Veronica. I don't know anything for

sure yet. I'm merely guessing because the radiology department is taking forever to get back to me. Rocco tried to tell me it doesn't mean anything terrible, but I still have a gut feeling. This has been such a crazy situation from the beginning. I'm not sure what to think."

"I don't blame you for being scared. I went through something similar when Remy was a baby. Rick was deployed overseas, and I got scary results back on my Pap smear. They thought I had cervical cancer. I didn't want Remy to be an only child. I had to do all these follow-up exams toting a baby in my arms. I was a basket case because I thought I would have to get a hysterectomy and face cancer all by myself while raising an infant. I was beside myself with grief and fear."

"What happened?"

"That's when I got a lesson in the world of false positives. Before then, I had no idea medical exams could be wrong. Lucky for me, I was one of those women who got a false positive result when everything was perfectly fine. Rick and I were afraid to trust the negative test results for a while. Even after he returned stateside, it took us a while to have enough faith to get pregnant with Rocco."

"I'm glad everything worked out for you. At the moment, I'm numb with fear. I haven't even told my parents what's going on because I'm not even sure what to say. They are not particularly supportive of what I have decided to do with my life and I have a feeling that in their minds, breast cancer would turn out to be my fault too."

"You never know. This might be the perfect opportunity for you to mend fences with your family."

"I really should. If this turns out to be what I think it is, I might not have much time left."

"Don't let Rocco hear you talk like that. Even if the worst is true, and you have breast cancer, survival rates are much higher these days than they used to be. You are young and strong! Look at it this way; because you helped your neighbor out, you caught it early — way early!"

I walk over and give Veronica a hug as tears flow down my face. "Thank you so much. I needed to hear that. I've been turning this over in my head so many times trying to figure out 'Why me?' I guess I forget millions of other women face breast cancer and beat it. I can do this. I can be one more."

"That's the spirit! Now, I have to figure out the sides for dinner. Do you prefer potato salad or pasta salad?"

"I am a potato salad kinda gal."

"Pickles or no pickles?"

"Pickles! Is there any other kind?"

"See? I knew my son had great taste in women! Would you like to help me put it together?"

"Sure, I'm not Julia Child or anything, but I like to cook."

I clutch Rocco's hand as we weave through the crowd in the big oversized barn. I glance up at the banner hanging above the stage which reads Locate My Heart. "We've covered several stories involving them at *Word Soup*. The story of Toby Payne was simply haunting. I can't get it out of my head. Can you imagine being kidnapped when you're just a kid and waiting years to be found? I would've lost hope. What happened to him was a miracle. The folks at Locate My Heart are miracle workers."

"I don't think Toby would disagree with you. It might surprise you to know he is one of your biggest fans," Rocco responds as he looks down at me and grins.

"No way! You're making that up!"

"I'm serious. He was teasing me because he works for a company who helps locate missing people and people who have been victims of identity theft. He told me he expected it to be a much bigger challenge. Toby never expected me to hire him to find someone he was already following on social media. He's probably here tonight. His brother is engaged to the director of Locate My Heart. Would you like to meet Toby?"

"I don't know. Would he think it's weird that I know about his story? I feel a bit like an online stalker."

"With all the media attention Toby's story received nationally, he's pretty used to people being curious about it. As long as you don't put your reporter hat on and grill him about the past, I'm pretty sure he'd be cool with it."

I giggle. "Okay, I'll try to tamp down my natural tendencies and not be nosy." Rocco chooses a table near the stage and pulls out a chair for me. Just then, a group of musicians climbs the stairs to the stage. The entertainment beat is not my thing, but even I know who these people are. "Oh my gosh, Rocco! These are not just any old coffee shop singers — that's Aidan O'Brien, Tasha and Jude, and Mindy Whitaker. I did some research into Mindy for a story on the use of psychics in solving crimes. I became a huge fan of her music in the process."

"If you're a fan of her music, you'll be even a bigger fan of her as a person. She is extraordinary."

A young guy with dark hair approaches our table. "Jigger, jig, jig, you mind if I sit here? You guys have jigger, jig, jig, great access to the stage and I have big plans."

I gesture toward the table. "Sure, there is plenty of room."

Rocco stands up and greets him. "Elijah, how is your dad? That was a pretty nasty fall Seth took."

"He's fine. Jigger, jig, jig, Dad was just embarrassed he fell while he was transferring into the shower. Thanks for not making a big deal out of it."

Rocco shrugs. "We rescue people from situations like his all the time, it's our job. It really isn't a problem. I'm glad he wasn't hurt. So, tell us about your big plans."

Elijah pulls out a chair, shrugs off his backpack, and sets it down on the ground. He nods toward me and sticks out his hand. "Jigger, jig, jig, hi I'm Elijah Fisher. I write books."

Belatedly, I remember to close my mouth before I reply, "Um … I know. I've read some of them. As a Japanese-American who was adopted by Caucasian parents, I was bullied a lot as a kid. *Behind Glass Bars* profoundly spoke to me. I'm Mallory Yoshida, by the way. I write too, but not the way you do. I am a journalist. I cover the crime beat."

Elijah blushes slightly. "Jigger, jig, jig, thank you so much. That book changed my life in many ways, jigger, jig, jig. It was also the first time I met Mindy. Someday, when I'm not a nervous wreck, remind me to tell you how my — hopefully — soon to be fiancé saved my family's life."

"I covered a little of that story for *Word Soup*, but I

would love some inside insight."

Rocco chuckles, "Hey, Ms. Reporter, I think you overlooked the biggest scoop. If I didn't miss Elijah's point, I think he's planning to pop the question tonight, right?"

This time, I'm the one whose face heats. "Oh my gosh! I'm so sorry! I stomped all over your news. Occupational hazard I guess, I tend to focus on all the gory stuff. Congratulations!"

Before Elijah can respond, his attention is drawn to the stage. He sits transfixed as Mindy walks toward him. Her hair is braided artfully to keep her wild blonde hair out of her face while the rest flows in riotous curls down her shoulders. She is wearing a lavender gauze dress which is tied at the waist with a leather belt. She looks like a forest nymph from a fairytale. When she reaches our table, she leans down and kisses him. "How did it sound from over here? I feel like the mic isn't picking up my acoustic guitar very well."

"Jigger, jig, jig, I'd like to say you sound gorgeous as usual, but I think you have a point. You're being drowned out a little by Jude," Elijah says before he enthusiastically returns her kiss.

Waiting for the moment of intimacy to pass, I add. "I've never heard you live, but you sounded pretty good to me."

It's almost as if Mindy didn't notice me sitting at the table and she has the oddest reaction I've ever seen. I'm used to people not knowing what to make of my race in small-town Oregon — but her reaction is downright strange. She studies me for a couple of seconds and then sways on her feet as the blood drains out of her face.

Elijah helps her sit in a chair next to me and pours her a glass of ice water from the pitcher sitting in the middle of the table. "Breathe through it, jigger, jig, jig," he murmurs in her ear. "Information is power, remember?"

Mindy draws in a shuddering breath. "I know. But sometimes I just hate what I see."

Just then, the full weight of what Mindy is saying hits me. All the parts of the puzzle start to fall into place. I gasp and then pull in a deep breath. "Mindy, I know what you do. I've studied your gift and what it's meant for law enforcement. I can tell from your expression whatever you see about my future is devastating. I also know I'm expecting some results from an ultrasound and follow-up mammogram. It doesn't take a rocket scientist to figure out those two things are probably related. Rocco brought me here tonight because I was going crazy waiting for information from the hospital. If you have news for me, I welcome it, even if it's bad. Not knowing is absolutely killing me."

Mindy's eyes widen with surprise. "I have to be honest. That's not the reaction I usually get when people learn about what I do. I wish I had better news. From what I see, you're in for a fight. Breast cancer is not common in people your age, but it does happen. There's a part of this that makes little sense. It looks like your diagnosis will actually help you in your job. I wish I could spell it out more clearly, but my gift doesn't work that way. I see bits and pieces. I see a battle, but I don't see you losing the war — if that makes any sense. You've got lots of people on your team." Mindy stands up to leave.

"Thanks Mindy. I appreciate your honesty, even though it's hard to tell people bad news." I rise to give her a long hug.

As she pulls away, she adds one last remark, "I'm adopted too. So, I understand that it can be complicated, but your adoptive parents should be on your team."

"You're not the first person to tell me that recently. I'll work on building some bridges."

"I'm so sorry I couldn't give you happy news. I've got to go get ready for the concert. I hope you and Rocco enjoy it. I wish our meeting could have gone differently."

"Surprisingly, I'm not all that upset with how it went. Now that I know, I can start to make some plans. Thank you."

Chapter Nine

Rocco

Mindy's spontaneous announcement may have brought a sense of peace to Mallory, but I'm not sure it did the same for me. I watch my date quietly as she is enthralled with Mindy and Joe Summers' performance of *Silver Bells*. No one seems to mind that it's nowhere near Christmas as everyone listens to the beautiful, chart-topping duet. All I can think about is what Mallory will actually be doing at Christmas time. I've seen what radiation and chemotherapy does to patients and it's not pretty.

After the thunderous applause dies down, Mindy clears her throat. "I'd like to call my little brother, Charlie, and my boyfriend, Elijah, to the stage."

Elijah looks dazed. "Jigger, jig, jig, this wasn't part of the plan," he mutters.

I clap him on the back as I hold up my camera. "It's okay, we've got you covered. Just roll with it."

"I don't do well with unexpected changes, jigger, jig, jig," he wheezes.

Mallory touches him on the forearm as he walks by. "I understand. I'm like that too, but you've got this. Whatever you do, she'll be enchanted."

Elijah looks over his shoulder and mouths, "Thanks."

Mallory moves her chair closer to mine and leans into my side as she rests her head on my shoulder. "This is going to be romantic," she whispers as she surreptitiously positions her camera on the table so she can record the encounter.

The crowd laughs as Charlie bolts across the room and bounds onto the stage. Elijah is a little more reluctant as he climbs the stairs and stands next to Mindy. He shields his eyes against the stage lights before he puts his arm around her waist.

Mindy addresses the crowd, "I bet you're wondering why I called two of my favorite guys up on stage." Charlie nods vigorously, and the crowd laughs. "Well, I'm so proud of them I couldn't keep it to myself any longer. I just wanted to tell you "Reading Is for Life" has reached out and they want to feature *CJ's World* written by Elijah Fischer and illustrated by Charlie Whitaker in their catalog."

Charlie looks up at his sister in shock. "Our book? In those catalogs that go out to all the school kids? Like all the kids everywhere, all around the world could order it?"

Mindy nods. "Isn't that cool? You know what's even better? They want to talk to you and Elijah about having Jiggernut Publishing produce a whole series of CJ books."

"You mean we might do more than one book?

Awesome!" He turns toward Elijah. "Can we?"

Elijah still appears to be processing the news, but he leans forward and says, "Seems like we have an audience to please. Jigger, jig, jig, I've learned to never disappoint book lovers. It looks like we need to do some serious brainstorming."

"Lucky for you, I brought some paper tonight," Charlie says as he dashes off stage.

Mindy chuckles and shakes her head. "My little brother never goes anywhere at a normal pace. I'm told I was a lot like him as a kid. Anyway, I hope you enjoyed hearing my exciting news. I'm sure you all came to hear my Uncle Aidan sing. As the saying goes, the show must go on."

Elijah is still standing quietly beside Mindy trying not to let his nerves show. After a few moments she looks up at him and laughs. "I love you — but if you don't want to sing backup, you might want to go sit down."

He steps away from the microphone and clears his throat. "Jigger, jig, jig, in a minute. We need to talk."

"Here?" Mindy squeaks as she points to the audience.

"That's the plan, jigger, jig, jig."

Mindy looks dubious. "Are you sure?"

Elijah nods. "Jigger, jig, jig, I've never been so sure of anything in my life. As your friends and family know, it is virtually impossible to surprise you — but I'm going to try."

"Elijah … are you going to make me cry?" Mindy covers her mouth with her hand.

"Jigger, jig, jig, it's a distinct possibility." He gets

down on one knee.

"I don't even know if my Papa is here to see this," Mindy cries as she wipes tears from her cheeks with the back of her hand.

"No worries, Mindy Mouse," Denny Ashley answers from the back of the room. "You know your grandma and I wouldn't miss one of your concerts for the world."

Elijah removes a ring from his pocket and holds it out towards Mindy. "Mindy Joe Whitaker, jigger, jig, jig, I've been in love with you almost from the moment I met you all those years ago. Jigger, jig, jig, I probably wasn't anything close to your dream guy. I was awkward, shy and a little funny looking. I had braces, glasses, and I talked funny. Not only that — I randomly hit myself, made funny faces and counted strange things. Sadly, not much has changed. Jigger, jig, jig. The braces came off, I wear contact lenses and I have a better hairstylist. Even so, I still have Tourette's syndrome. Even with the new medication, I still have tics which make me strike myself and, jigger, jig, jig, blurt gibberish."

Mindy reaches out and ruffles his hair. "I don't mind. All that doesn't matter. It's not as if I don't have my own quirks."

"I know. That's what makes our love story truly extraordinary. Mindy Jo Whitaker, will you marry me and love me until the end of time and until all of our memories have faded into yesterdays?"

Mindy nods mutely and signs yes in American Sign Language as she holds her hand out for Elijah to slide the ring on.

Aidan O'Brien who had been watching the whole event unfold from his perch on the stage leans into his microphone and explains, "For those of you not fluent in sign language, the little girl I watched grow up and consider to be my honorary niece just said yes to the man of her dreams. I couldn't be happier."

"Jigger, jig, jig, before I put this on your finger, I want you to look at it," Elijah says to Mindy as he kisses her gently. "Jigger, jig, jig. Thank you for saying yes. I know it's a cliché, but you've made me the happiest man on the planet."

Mindy takes the ring from Elijah and looks at it again. "How did you do this? It looks almost exactly like my bracelet!" Turning to the audience, Mindy explains, "When I was adopted, my dad gave me and my baby sister bracelets promising to love us until the stars fall from the sky. It's the same promise he made our mom when he asked her to marry him." She holds up her arm for the audience to see. "I've cherished this bracelet since that day. The only time I've ever had it off is when I had to have my wisdom teeth out."

"I know how much traditions, love and commitment mean to you. Jigger, jig, jig, look inside the ring."

Mindy turns the ring in her hand and examines the inside of the band. When she sees what's printed there, she dissolves into tears. "Darn it! You're making me ugly cry in front of all these people." She shields her eyes against the stage lights as she looks out into the audience. "Daddy, you were right. Elijah is perfect for me. He understands everything. Thank you for not letting him give up on me when I was pushing him away. I know all of you in the audience can't see what this says, but Elijah was thoughtful enough to carry on our family tradition. The engraving reads 'UNTIL'." She hands the ring back to Elijah. "I will happily wear this ring until the end of time when there are no more tomorrows."

The audience erupts in applause as Elijah and Mindy seal their engagement with a passionate kiss. Aidan O'Brien clears his throat as he announces, "I'm going to sing some corny love songs as I give my backup singer a little while to collect herself and show off her ring to her family. Isn't love grand? Congratulations Mindy Mouse!"

Mindy collects herself and wipes away tears. "By the way, the perfect engagement gift for Elijah and me would be a donation to Locate My Heart. It's a charity that means a lot to both of us."

After Elijah and Mindy go backstage, Mallory shuts off her camera. "What an amazing love story! You told me Mindy was phenomenal. You weren't kidding. I think Elijah is cool too. I thought so when I read his book a few years ago — but he's even more impressive in person. I'm glad they're together. I don't understand everything there is to know about Mindy's gift, but it has to be exhausting. I bet Elijah understands a lot of what she goes through."

"My friend Jaxson is married to her aunt. Donda says Mindy is much happier since Elijah came back into her life. Apparently, Mindy has always been the kind of person who carries the weight of the world on her shoulders. Elijah helps share the load. He's actually quite funny if you can get him to let down his guard around you."

Mallory grabs my phone and flips through the pictures I took throughout the whole proposal. She sighs wistfully. "This was so perfect. If I can beat the whole cancer thing, I want to find a guy who will do something like this for me. I don't want extravagant trips, cruises, or a proposal in the middle of an NFL game or anything. I want someone who knows me well enough to know that a single word engraved inside of a ring would make me never want to take it off."

Mallory's words remind me that whatever I have with her is based on a very flimsy construct. Although my feelings are quite real, the whole premise is artificial. I'm just pretending to be her husband for now. Somehow, I keep forgetting that I'm not the real thing. I'm not even really her boyfriend. I swallow hard before I carefully choose my words. "I hope whoever you find makes all your dreams come true because it's not *if* you beat cancer, but *when* you beat cancer. I have no doubt we'll be throwing a party when you are five years cancer free and again when ten years rolls around."

"Do you truly think so?" Mallory asks. "I'm almost afraid to hope for anything."

"One of the things we learn as paramedics is that at least part of the outcome is based on mental outlook. Whether it's faith in a higher power or good old-fashioned hope that things will get better, I don't know. But, I do know believing in a positive outcome does make a huge difference. As your dedicated, pretend husband I'll be by your side to cheer you on every step of the way. You can beat a few mutant cells, you are a warrior!"

"I can see your mom's enthusiasm is contagious. Veronica gave me almost an identical speech this afternoon. Did you guys practice together or something?" Mallory jokes with a tight smile.

"Actually, we didn't — but like I said, my mom is very persuasive. She is also a very powerful ally. If she is in your corner, watch out. She will move everything in her path to get her way. Lord help the person who crosses her."

"Maybe we should sic her on the hospital if they don't hurry up and get the results back to me. I'm tired of waiting."

"That would be an interesting strategy for sure. But I'm not sure we are ready to go nuclear on the hospital just yet. I'll ask Jaxson to poke around and see if he can figure out what's taking them so long."

"I'd appreciate it. I'm tired of waiting around. I want to make plans — even if they aren't the plans I had hoped for."

As I'm walking in the door to go on shift, my phone rings. "This is Rocco," I answer without looking.

"Well, after all that time waiting, the call was quite anti-climactic," Mallory declares abruptly, without preamble. "They want me to make an appointment for a biopsy. Maybe it just seems less dramatic because I already knew what the news would be because I found out from Mindy."

"Aww, I'm sorry Mal. I was hoping Mindy would be wrong, although I knew the odds of that were slim. Word on the street is she's never, ever been wrong. Are you okay?"

Mallory sighs. "Yes and no. I thought I was coping pretty well — but then Edna came over and saw I'd been crying. She wanted to know why. I couldn't very well lie to her. Now, Edna blames herself for the fact that she tried to guilt me into getting a mammogram. You know, back in the old days mammograms were a lot more powerful and her generation had the misconception that the tests themselves cause the cancer. That's not true. The whole conversation was a disaster. Edna thinks she caused all of it."

"Oh geez, I'm sorry. That's rough. Sometimes, there's just no talking people out of their belief systems either. Maybe I can have a conversation with her and explain it."

Before Mallory can answer, a call goes out over the intercom system and over our radios. Since I am still in the vehicle bay, the sound echoes everywhere. "I'm sorry, a call just came in. I've got to go. I'll try to call on my lunch hour."

"Oh, I'm sorry! I didn't realize you were at work. Real quick — they offered me Tuesday or Friday in two weeks, which is better for you?"

"Definitely Tuesday," I answer. "If I catch some time over lunch, I'll call you."

I put my phone in my pocket and lean against the truck as I try to collect my thoughts. Raylene takes one look at me and asks, "You look stressed. Need me to drive? Let me guess, Chevy did something crazy again? Did you have to take him to the vet?"

I shrug. "You can if you want. My day is off to a rough start." Chevy has had more than his fair share of trips to the local vet. He is not the picture of grace. I shake my head as my expression grows sober. "Unfortunately, my friend's cancer diagnosis was confirmed this morning. She has to go in for a biopsy to see which stage of breast cancer she has."

"I've been through this before. As much as it sucks, a biopsy doesn't mean she has cancer yet. They could still rule it out."

"I sorta doubt that'll happen at this stage," I argue.

"What happened to you?"

"Oh, my mom didn't catch her breast cancer until she was late stage IV. So, she passed away when I was in high school."

I flinch as she shares her story. Raylene notices my reaction before I could cover it with something more socially acceptable. "Sorry, I guess I just wanted to remind you that not everybody's story is the same. Everyone's fight is individual to them — your friend's biopsy might show something, or it might not. Wherever you and your friend go, people will tell you about the most heroic cancer legend whether it be real or fictitious. Other people feel compelled to tell you the goriest, most horrendous battle with cancer they've ever heard of without regard to your own pain and suffering."

I bristle at Raylene's brutally honest assessment. "Why do people feel they have the right to be that way? Don't they understand cancer is difficult enough on its own?"

"I think there are a lot of people who are trying to be helpful. As for the other folks, I truly don't know. Maybe they're trying to get sympathy points for having the worst sob story. I never understood it even when I had to go into foster care."

"So, you might have already figured this out. Mallory is more than just my friend — or I would like her to be when this is all said and done. How can I avoid being one of those people who fall into the jerk category?"

"Don't assume that just because you're a paramedic with medical knowledge you know what's going on. Ask questions — but be willing to listen to the answers. Try not to make her entire world about cancer. It's so isolating when everything in your entire universe is about killing a few cells in your boobs. When you have cancer, you lose your sense of identity and purpose. You can help her keep that. Help her feel beautiful even when she's hanging her head over a dishpan and her hair falls out in the shower."

"Mallory has beautiful hair — but if she loses it because of chemotherapy, I won't fall out of love with her. That would be ludicrous."

"It's one thing for us to sit here and calmly discuss it. It's a completely different thing to live through it. You guys are in a brand-new relationship. She may not even trust her ability to keep your attention in sexy little outfits, high heels and full makeup. She may fear she has no chance if she has to have a mastectomy and chemotherapy and radiation."

"Oh, for Pete's sake, of all the things for Mallory to worry about — that's insane. I don't care about any of that stuff. I just want her to live."

"Rocco, I know all that about you because I've been your partner for a long time. Mallory just met you. You need to have a heart-to-heart conversation and let her know what you're thinking. She can't read your mind. It might make you both feel better about the situation."

CHAPTER TEN

MALLORY

ROCCO WALKS UP TO the table of the little bistro a few blocks from my office where I agreed to meet him for lunch and pulls me up to a standing position. He acts like he hasn't seen me in months as he drops a passionate kiss on my lips. When we finally break apart, I have to take a moment to catch my breath. You'd never guess we had a family dinner over at Edna's house only three nights ago. It was a blast retelling the story of Mindy's engagement and the family gathering we were invited to afterwards at a local truck stop. I was shocked at how normal Aidan O'Brien and his whole crew were. I suppose I expected they would be changed by stardom and somehow different from the rest of us. Yet, I found I have a lot in common with Mindy's friend, Madison, who used to be a journalist and her grandmother Gwendolyn who is a lung cancer survivor.

I realize I must have completely spaced out during my conversation with Rocco when he snaps his fingers in front of my face. "I know I told you I have a reputation for being a great kisser, but I've never had it render a person completely catatonic before. Do I need to kiss you again to reverse some sort of spell?" he quips.

I shake my head as if to release some invisible spell. "No, I'm just stressed, and I got lost in my thoughts of the other night."

Rocco winks at me. "I hear you. When I think about that night, I get distracted too. I get lost in memories of how perfectly you fit in my arms and how I never wanted to let you go."

I groan in frustration. "I wish I could go back to that night. If everything is so perfect, why is there all this paperwork? It never seems to end."

"What's up?" He examines the piles of paperwork spread out on the table in front of me.

I throw up my hands in frustration. "I don't even know how to fill half of this stuff out. You know, I could eliminate a bunch of these if you were actually my husband."

"Sounds good," he says as he sits down at the table.

"Be serious! I'm just saying for a system who gave you my medical records on a whim, they make it remarkably hard for me to give them to you on purpose."

"Who said I wasn't being serious? The way we met may have been a bit unorthodox, but I click with you on levels I haven't connected with anyone else — ever. Is it so bad that I wish our pretend relationship was actually the real thing?"

I flush deep red and have to fan myself. "Honestly, I thought it was just me. At night, I dream we're a normal family. It seems so real, I'm disappointed when you're not there when I wake up."

"We can work on changing your fantasies to reality, anytime you say the word," Rocco offers with a wink.

You have no idea how much I wish I could make all this go away by merely uttering a few magic words. But I don't think that'll work. I point to another stack of papers. "Even if I ignore the paperwork about you, this is about my medical history. You know what? I know nothing about the medical history of Mallory Edmondson, Nariko Yoshida, Mallory Yoshida or whatever the heck you want to call me. It doesn't matter because either way I have no idea who I was before I was adopted or where I came from. It's all a mystery."

"Nariko is your real name?" Rocco asks with a quizzical look.

"Nariko Yoshida is the name written on my adoption papers. I was raised as Mallory Edmondson. My father's name is Edward Edmondson, the Second. My mother is Rosalind Edmondson. When my family practically disowned me over my decision to move to the West Coast and pursue journalism, I went back to my birth name to gain a sense of identity. To be honest, it was a way to hurt them because I felt abandoned. I kept the name Mallory because it was my grandmother's middle name and she always supported my dreams."

A family with a bunch of noisy, active kids sits down at the two tables next to us. With a concerned expression, Rocco looks around. "Do you have to go back to work?"

"Technically? No, I don't. I'm on indefinite medical leave until I feel well enough to come back. Andre's exact instructions were to 'Take a couple days to get your life together before it gets crazy. Don't worry about your stupid job.' I only came to work because I can't stand the quiet of my own thoughts. I'm driving myself crazy."

Rocco stands up and walks behind me as he massages my neck. "You won't be alone. I'll be there with you. Let's take all this back to your place where we can tackle it together, okay?"

"You're like magic. How do you always make things better?" I lean my head against his forearm.

"I guess I was just born to be a Mallory soother," he quips.

"That's a very good thing. I have the feeling that skill will be in great demand soon."

Rocco leans back in the kitchen chair. "This sandwich is the best thing I've eaten in a while."

"Don't thank me. The tomatoes are from Edna's garden. I wouldn't eat half as well as I do without her help."

"I'll be sure to thank her," Rocco says as he wipes his face with a paper towel.

"Edna loves you, you know? You made her feel so much better about what lies ahead for me. She was beginning to think my funeral might be tomorrow — but she's better now. She doesn't talk like it's her fault anymore. Although, she is knitting me a blanket for chemotherapy."

"Edna is a good lady. She reminds me of my own grandma." After Rocco takes his dishes over to the sink and washes his hands, he returns to the table where we have all the paperwork arranged in several stacks. He points to one stack. "Okay, I've got all the release forms filled out so I can talk to the doctors about your case even if they figure out I'm not really your husband. I found your living will in your paperwork, so all of that is together."

"How did you do it so quickly? Those forms were making me dizzy."

"I think my job gives me an advantage. I push paperwork around all day. I'm used to what it looks like."

I walk over to the table and pick up a folder. "What am I going to do about this one? They're asking a bunch of questions about my family. First, it's all about family history. I know nothing, really."

"I'm sure it's not the end of the world. Tons of people are adopted."

"Even if I figure that part out, they want to know about emergency contacts. Should I use my adoptive family? They haven't spoken to me in a few years. I suppose I could use Edna, but I hate to because I don't want to put any more stress on her. I could involve Andre but that's not exactly appropriate since he's my employee. I don't have a lot of friends in Oregon —" I confess as my voice breaks. I haven't even gotten to the hard stuff yet, and this is already starting to take an emotional toll on me.

"I understand this is tough to hear because of all the stuff you've gone through with your parents. It might be time for you to reach out to them. If I were a parent, I would be devastated if my child was sick and I didn't know."

"I know. I've turned that thought over and over in my head since you first came to me with my medical records. But I keep getting hung up on the same problem. How do you restart a conversation after more than half a decade? I don't know what to say."

"I guess if it were me I'd start with the basics. 'I love you.' 'I miss you.' 'I'm scared.' Or, 'I need you'. Honesty generally works the best."

"You make it sound so easy. What if they hate me? What if they never want to talk to me again? What if they don't care if I have cancer?"

Rocco wraps his arms around me from behind and whispers in my ear. "What if they do? What if the only thing keeping them from picking up the phone are the very same fears you're having? What if they can't find the words either? You need to make the call. It's important."

I turn and bury my face in his chest. "I'm scared."

"I know, Mal. That's why we're going to do this together. Grab your phone."

I reach behind me and pick my phone up off the table. Before I can blink, Rocco scoops me off my feet and carries me over to the couch. He puts his feet up on the coffee table and cuddles me on his lap. "Comfy?" he asks.

I nod as I pull up my dad's number in my phone. My hands are trembling so much I can barely hold my phone. Rocco strokes my back. "You can do this."

When a familiar voice answers the phone, I have to clear my throat a couple of times before I can form words. "Hi Mom, is Dad in the office today?"

I place the phone on speaker phone so Rocco can hear my mom say, "Oh goodness! Mallory is that really you?"

"Yes, Mom it's me. Do you think Dad would be willing to talk to me? Or is he still angry?"

"Why would you have such a crazy notion? Of

course your dad wants to talk to you. He waits every year on his birthday, Christmas and on Father's Day for you to call, but you never do. You never call on Mother's Day either."

"Mom, Dad said if I came to Portland to go to school, I might as well be dead to him because I didn't want to be a dentist."

"That's why you moved all the way across the United States and changed your name? For something your father said after the Celtics lost in the playoffs and he lost a bundle. Honey, your father was three sheets to the wind and not responsible for anything he said for several days. I finally kicked his butt out of the house and made him stay at a hotel because he was driving me crazy."

"I tried to talk to him for months after the big argument. Dad wouldn't talk to me or apologize. He just insisted he was right, and I was making all the wrong moves. I figured you both hated me and were sorry you adopted me in the first place."

"Oh honey, nothing could be further from the truth. Your father was devastated when he drove you away. You know how he is. I couldn't really pick sides. Anyway, he's just finishing up with the patient. Oh, just a second, I see the door opening right now. I'll try to catch him."

"Mom, when you put him on the phone, please stay on the line. I need to speak to you both."

"Sounds serious. You're not dying or anything are you?"

"It's complicated. I'd rather explain it just once. Can you get Dad on the line?" I plead as I lose my nerve. The phone clicks and music starts to play. I grimace as I recognize the same hold music my parents used to loop when I worked in the office as a teenager. I wonder if they're using the same outdated computer systems and filing systems too.

"Doesn't sound like they hate you," Rocco murmurs against my temple.

I shake my head. "It doesn't."

Abruptly, my phone clicks and I hear my dad's upper-crust accent. "I trust you haven't waited this long to go to the dentist."

"Edward! Knock it off. Mallory is finally calling home and it's your fault she hasn't called. Show some grace and manners, please."

"It's all right, Mom. As a matter of fact, I have been exercising excellent oral hygiene. At my last dental checkup, I had no cavities. My new dentist is very impressed with my protocol."

"What should I even call you? Is it Mallory or Nariko — or do you go by something else completely different by now?"

"Edward Edmonds, behave yourself! You know very well what your daughter calls herself; you follow her blog every single day. Stop being an obnoxious pill! If you don't, I'll kick you off this phone call and talk to our daughter myself."

"It's okay, Mom. Maybe I'm to blame too. Perhaps I should have asked more questions and not jumped to so many conclusions. But, I have a bigger fight on my hands now."

"Oh my gosh, I knew it. You *are* dying," my mom gasps.

"I don't think it's quite that dire yet. But all

indications are I have breast cancer. I have to go in for a biopsy on Tuesday. I've already had an ultrasound and a second mammogram. It looks pretty conclusive. I am petrified because I don't even have health insurance. The company I work for is just a small startup and can't afford to offer it. I make too much money to qualify for help from the government. So, I'm on my own."

My dad sighs heavily. "You were always the most confoundingly stubborn child. Why didn't you call us earlier? Did it ever occur to you that I am a doctor and before your mother gave up her career to help me run my practice, she was a nurse at a hospital? You have had health insurance — the most Cadillac of policies — on you since the day you came into our lives. We continue to pay premiums every month. Because we never believed you would stay gone. I'm sorry that whatever I said to you upset you. Your mother tried to tell me years ago I should apologize. I simply never believed you would leave over a few poorly chosen words. I figured maybe you no longer wanted to be an Edmondson. After all, you changed your name. Maybe you didn't want anything to do with us at all. Obviously, you know how to work a telephone because you called today. You could've done it much sooner."

"Edward, you are being totally unfair, telephones work both directions, you know. We could have just as easily called Mallory. She has birthdays and celebrates Christmas and Thanksgiving too."

"I wasn't the one who left. Mallory did," my dad argues stubbornly.

Rocco leans forward and talks into the phone, "With all due respect sir, your daughter is due to go under the knife and find out life altering news in about thirty-six hours. Is this really what you want your last conversation to be about?"

"Who are you?" my dad snaps at Rocco.

"I am Rocco Pierce. I am a friend of Mallory's. I care for her very much and I want to make sure this process goes as smoothly for her as possible. As a paramedic, I know that patients do well when they have positive family interactions. Would it be possible for one or both of you to be around for Mallory after surgery?"

I look at Rocco as if he's grown another head. At the moment, it's not even clear my parents and I can have a civil conversation from more than three thousand miles apart. I don't know what would happen if you put us in the same room together.

"Edward, I don't know who this gentleman is. But he's right. Are you going to let your pride get in the way again? It's been years since we've seen Mallory and now she's gravely ill. She needs us. What good does it do for us to hire partners in this practice if we never go on vacation? Let's go before it's too late."

"Where would we stay, Rosalind? You know I don't do well with spur-of-the-moment plans."

"You can stay at my house. I have a lovely guest room."

"How can you afford a house with a guest room if you can't afford health insurance benefits?" My dad presses.

"Look, it's a really long story and when you get here, I may feel up to telling you. I'll send Mom an email with all the information about how to get to my house. I'll figure out a way to get you picked up at the Portland airport so you don't have to get a taxi. It might be my friend Rocco or my assistant Andre from the newspaper."

I hear my mom take a shuddering breath. "Mallory, I'm very sad for the circumstances, but I'm so happy you called me. I've missed you so much over the past few years. I can't even put it into words. I'm excited to see you. I'll work on getting tickets right away. Hopefully we can fly out in the next day or so. I want to have some time to spend with you before your surgery. I love you honey, don't forget that. I'm sorry you ever thought otherwise."

My eyes tear up and I have to swallow hard a few times before I can answer. "I love you guys too. I can't wait to see you. I've missed you. I can't tell you how glad I am you don't hate me. I was so scared to call."

In the background, I hear the office phones go crazy. My mom groans out loud. "I swear they haven't been this busy all week."

"It's all right, Mom. Take care of business. I'll be in touch, I promise. I'll send you all of my contact information so you can make travel arrangements. I will see you guys in a couple of days."

Rocco squeezes my shoulder gently and I take a deep breath before I whisper, "I love you both so much. I'm glad I called."

Tears are streaming down my face as I hang up the phone. For several minutes, Rocco simply holds me as I weep. Years of pent-up emotions pour out of me.

I cry for so long, I start to hiccup. Rocco grabs a throw pillow and pops it behind me as he shimmies out from under me and places me gently on the couch and props me up. "I'll be right back."

He hands me the remote. "Edna tells me you have a weakness for Meg Ryan movies."

"She wasn't supposed to tell you about my addiction to 80s RomComs. I'm supposed to be a hardened, steely crime reporter," I protest through an awkward combination of hiccups and sniffles.

"We'll talk about what I watch in a minute," Rocco promises as he rushes toward my kitchen.

I flip through the channels and find a rerun of *Hope Floats*. Even though I've seen the movie dozens of times, I choose it. It's appropriately mushy for my emotional state. At least if I can't stop crying, I can blame it on the sad movie.

When Rocco comes back in the room, he's got a tray full of junk food. He brought two kinds of Ben & Jerry's ice cream, a bowl of popcorn, a can of pretzels and a bag of potato chips. I look at him with a confused expression. "The magic ingredient isn't quite ready yet. By the way, awesome double boiler. I've always wanted a copper one."

His phone beeps and he dashes back to the kitchen. When he comes back, he's carrying my gravy boat. He opens my coat closet and grabs a TV tray we used the other day when Edna came over to play cards. He sets the gravy boat in the middle and runs back to my kitchen. When he returns, he has a stack of paper plates, a handful of plastic bowls, and a roll of paper towels.

I struggle to sit up. "I'm not even sure I want to know how many Burpees I'll have to do to cope with whatever you have planned."

Rocco hands me a paper towel to wipe my face. "It's simple. Chocolate sauce is the cure for everything."

"Not quite so simple. If it was, I wouldn't be having holes drilled in me."

"Okay, maybe it doesn't cure everything, but it makes it all a little easier to deal with."

"I thought that's what my friends Cherry Garcia and Chunky Monkey were for," I answer with a tearful grin.

"They are good — but nothing says they can't be made better with a little warm chocolate sauce. I'm going to get myself a bowl of ice cream with chocolate sauce right now. Would you like some?"

"Not right now. I want to know what you have planned for the chips, pretzels, and popcorn."

Rocco shoots me a shocked expression worthy of a cartoon character. "You mean you haven't been introduced to the magic of salty and sweet?"

I wrinkle my nose. "Oh gross! Don't tell me you're planning to eat them together?"

"Don't knock it until you've tried it." Rocco digs a potato chip out of the bag and dips it in the chocolate. He holds it out for me to try. I'm hesitant at first. It occurs to me that I'm being ridiculous. Very soon, I'll have to take much bigger risks with him. I close my eyes and open my mouth like a baby bird.

I hear him break off a small piece and place it on my tongue. As I process all the tastes and textures, I realize it's not nearly as terrible as I expected. In fact, I actually like it. Rocco must be able to read the surprise on my face.

"It's good, isn't it? I told you you'd like it."

"You were right. You were right about a lot of stuff. I'm glad you convinced me to call my parents. Can you believe the whole fight was because my dad was frustrated because he lost money on a sports bet? All those years I lost with them — it's crazy. I thought they hated me. I won't get those years back. I may not have very many more years to live … and we were fighting over nothing. The whole thing is just stupid! I don't know if I should be relieved or just totally ticked off. Right now, I'm just sad. We may not get a second shot."

"I can't tell you how sorry I am about that. I know my relationship with my parents means the world to me. But some good things have happened because of your estrangement. You learned how to stand up for yourself — even when it meant facing dire consequences. You became a homeowner and the world's most supportive neighbor. You became a reporter with a mission to change the world and make a difference. People respect your reporting. You have fans all over, young and old — including your dad. I don't know if any of that would've happened if you hadn't been forced to struggle and make it on your own."

"Well, that's one way of looking at all the crap that's happened. I suppose you're one of those people who think if I do have cancer, have to chop my breasts off and lose all my hair that there's some grand meaning in it all."

Rocco puts down the ice cream he was dishing up as his expression grows fierce.

"Mallory, listen to me. I am not happy you're sick. But I am so grateful for Edna and her crazy plan to introduce you to a rich, successful doctor. I only wish this thing between us was real. If I had my way, you wouldn't be looking for your perfect guy after you beat cancer because that guy would be me."

I scoff. "Like I'll be in any shape to be looking for anybody. I'm going to look like some weird creature from a science fiction movie with no hair and no breasts who's about half as tall as a normal human being."

"I thought we already established height is no barrier between us. I'm serious when I say although I think your hair is beautiful, if you lost every strand of hair, I would still consider you the most extraordinarily beautiful woman I have ever met. As far as your breasts go, they're pretty — but they're not who you are. If you have to get rid of them to save your life, I wouldn't give them a second thought."

"We met by a cruel twist of fate. How do you know you want to give up your chance at a normal relationship for me? I might not survive this. You know that, right? Of course you know that! You're a paramedic. You see sick people all the time — people dying of cancer. You know what the end could be like."

"I'm not a doctor, but I know the odds are overwhelmingly in your favor. It's true, I haven't known you a long time. We didn't have the privilege of growing up together and hanging out at the mall, going to the movies or football games — although something tells me you were probably a band or choir geek."

"I played second chair flute."

"Even though I've only known you a couple of months, there isn't a part of me who wants to find anyone else. When I go to bed at night, I can't wait until the next time I see you again. When my phone rings, I hope it's you. If something awful happens at work, you're the first person I want to tell because I know you'll understand my pain."

"Wow! Did we accidentally become a real couple when we were pretending to be husband-and-wife? The timing sucks big time though. After Tuesday, I may look like a freak."

"Do you understand what I'm saying? To me it doesn't matter whether you lose your hair or your breasts. How you look doesn't change a thing about how I feel about you."

I lean across the table and kiss him gently. "How in the world did I ever get lucky enough to find a guy like you?"

Rocco winks. "Well, technically I found you."

"However it happened, I must've built up some mighty positive karma."

"That's what happens when you go to crazy extremes to make your elderly neighbors happy."

The CNA in charge of taking my vitals looks skeptically around the cramped room. My mom is still fussing with the blankets at my feet, but Edna gets the message. She walks over, carefully avoiding the machinery and cords with her cane as she bends over and kisses me on the cheek. "Hang in there. I'm going to spend the day cooking all your favorite foods. If you thought you were spoiled before, you have no idea what's coming."

"Edna, I may not feel up to eating for a while. I've heard anesthesia can make you nauseous."

My dad interrupts my conversation. "Nonsense Mallory, I did some reading on the plane. According to the medical journals, they might use a local anesthetic. You may not even be put to sleep for this procedure."

"Dad, I already spoke to the anesthesiologist. Based on where they have to take the biopsies, they plan to put me out — at least for a little while. They'll take a sample of my lymph nodes and do a core biopsy."

"How long before you know the results, honey?" my mom asks.

"The radiologist and the lab folks will be on hand to examine the samples and the images. If the results turn out to be positive for cancer, they will go ahead and do surgery. If it looks like my breast can be saved, they'll take the affected portion off during a lumpectomy. If it's extensive, they'll take both breasts in a full mastectomy."

My mom gasps. "Are you ready for all of that?"

Rocco reaches out and tucks a stray lock of hair back under the goofy little disposable hat they've already placed on my head as he brushes his knuckles down my cheek. He reaches out to grab my free hand which doesn't have an IV in it.

I shake my head. "No Mom, I'm not ready — cancer didn't really give me a choice. It'll be what it is. I've got a lot of people around me who care about what happens to me. That's about the best I can do under the circumstances."

Edna clears her throat. "Speaking as one of the people who cares about Mallory, I think we should get out of her hair so the medical staff can take care of her. Come on, Mr. and Mrs. Edmondson, let's grab some breakfast. It's going to be a long day."

Mom turns to me. "How will we know what's happening with you?"

"I programmed your numbers into Rocco's phone. As soon as he hears from the doctor, he'll keep you updated."

My mom walks over and gives me a big hug. She stands up and embraces Rocco too. "You promise to take good care of her?"

"I've been doing my best, Rosalind," Rocco responds.

My mom tears up. "I know. This is just so hard. It's the first time my baby has ever had surgery."

Edna puts her arm around my mom's waist as she walks her out of the room. "I know it's hard to see her hurting, but she's strong."

Rocco nods at my dad. "I'll call the minute I hear something. Go have yourself a nice breakfast. I'm far too nervous to eat. I'll stay here at the hospital."

My dad squeezes my toe as he clears his throat. "I better go. You know your mother, she gets lost in a heartbeat. She'll never find the car on her own."

"I'll be fine, Daddy," I promise as I close my eyes and fight back tears.

The CNA escorts my dad out of the room leaving only Rocco.

He dabs at my eyes with a Kleenex before he leans over and brushes a kiss across my lips. "Nariko, you are a warrior. Whatever this is, you will beat it. I'll be right by your side for the battle."

Two more nurses come into the room and introduce themselves. At this point, my pulse is pounding so badly in my ears I can't hear their perky introductions.

As I am being wheeled away, I squeeze Rocco's hand. "Of all the guys on the planet, I'm glad you turned out to be my husband."

CHAPTER ELEVEN

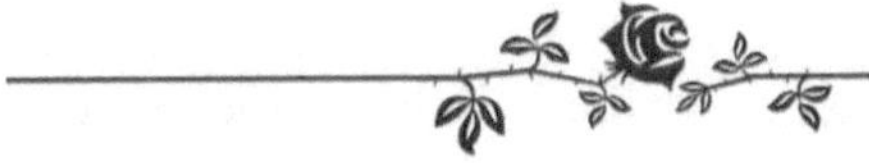

ROCCO

I'VE SAT IN PLENTY of waiting rooms during my career as a paramedic. I'm not one of those guys who could simply let all my patients go without a second thought. I often wait with family members to see how the questionable cases resolve. Those cases are tough, but nothing like this. I feel like a little piece of my heart is being chipped away with every tick of the clock. It doesn't help that I know the longer she stays under the knife, the more negative the outcome.

My stomach growls, reminding me it's been several hours since I've eaten. I receive a text message, but it's not from the hospital. It's from my friend, Tyler Colton, who works for the sheriff's office. I guess word gets around because he wants to know which waiting room I'm in. I get up and look around until I locate a room number and text it to him.

I sit back down and try to read a magazine, but my concentration is shot. The sound of the old-fashioned school clock on the wall drowns out all rational thought.

I'm surprised when I look up and see Tyler and his

wife, Heather. She's holding out a bag from her bakery. "I brought your usual plus a couple of fresh baked goodies. I thought you might be hungry. If you're anything like Ty, you've probably been worried sick and are too stressed to eat."

"Have you heard anything yet?" Tyler asks with a concerned expression.

"The doctor came out and updated me once. The biopsy was positive for cancer cells. Based on the samples they took, and the imaging, they feel they can contain it with just a lumpectomy. I guess it was incredible luck she had that spur-of-the-moment mammogram with Edna. There is evidence the cancer may be encroaching on her lymph nodes. — but just barely. They've tentatively categorized her as stage 1B. If her margins come back clean, she shouldn't need any radiation, only chemotherapy. It won't be easy, but it's all very treatable."

"How is the surprise reunion with her parents going?" Heather grimaces. "I know if that had happened with my family, I might have branded it almost as stressful as finding out I had breast cancer."

"Actually, I think that's the biggest surprise in all of this. It's going better than anyone expected. The whole thing seems to have sprung up around a series of complete misunderstandings rather than any real animosity. So, in a weird way the cancer may have turned out to be one of those blessings in disguise, as cliché as it sounds."

Tyler nods, "It's not the first time I've heard that. Jeff says his mom's cancer saved the relationship between his mom and his sister. So, good things can come out of terrible situations."

"Well, I'm hoping for an all-around miracle. Not only am I praying for the best outcome for Mallory's cancer, I'm hoping for a love story to spring up from all this mess. I met her because of this medical catastrophe and I fell in love with her despite of it. But I'm afraid she'll never be able to separate the two things. I don't want her to always associate me with the absolute worst news of her entire life — but I don't know how we'll ever get past that even once the initial crisis is over."

"Not to burst your bubble or anything buddy, but I think your woman will have much bigger issues on her mind than where or how she met you. When, how, or if you guys get your relationship together is kind of a back-burner topic at the moment. If you happen to get it sorted out, cool. If you don't, I wouldn't worry about it. She's got enormous stuff to deal with."

"I know. I feel guilty even thinking about it. I can't even picture my life without Mallory in it now. So, it's weird not to think about it, if you know what I mean."

Heather smiles sympathetically. "I understand exactly what you mean. I had known Ty for a long time, but around the time our relationship got serious, my grandma died. I couldn't believe I was falling in love during the saddest time of my life. It just seemed bizarre to me. When I realized Ty was exactly the kind of man Grandma Lydia would've wanted for me, I forgave myself for any awkward timing. Sometimes, what doesn't make sense to the outside world makes perfect sense to your heart."

I unwrap the sub sandwich and gratefully take a few bites. "You guys have been married for quite a while now, right?" I ask as I pause to take a drink of my bitter coffee I've been nursing for what seems like hours and it's cold as ice. "I guess that means you were able to work through your issues?"

Tyler nods. "The death of Heather's grandmother was only the beginning. I was not a huge hit with her parents and then there was the stress of opening Joy and Tiers."

Heather smirks. "I think you forgot the major event, Lieutenant Colonel Colton."

"No, I didn't forget," Tyler says ruefully. "I just try to block that part out. I hate how stressful my deployment was for you and our marriage."

"Wow! How did you guys keep your sanity and survive?"

"It wasn't easy. We just tried to focus on the bright side of things and the strength of our relationship. I won't lie and say it was easy. In fact, when Tyler left to report for duty, I was afraid maybe he'd given up on us."

I look at Tyler in utter disbelief. "Mr. Loyalty, Commitment and Service to Country?"

Ty shrugs. "I wasn't great about communicating what mattered to me."

Heather nods. "Back then, I wasn't too sure anybody would love me for me. I was convinced I was wholly unlovable. It took Ty years to fix the damage."

"Do you have any advice for me?" I ask.

Tyler looks at me solemnly. "No matter what the two of you face, it doesn't change why you fell in love with Mallory. She still is that person under all of her pain. Some days, it may be harder to find her. Just never forget to look."

Heather nods. "Remember, you're fighting cancer,

not each other. I know it seems obvious now, but when you're tired, stressed and nothing in your life seems normal, those lines can get a little blurred."

I stand up and give each of them a brief hug. "Thanks for stopping by. I appreciate the food and the pep talk. I needed them."

Heather hugs me back. "Don't worry about it. When Mallory feels better, we'll include her in the Girlfriend Posse. Gwendolyn has been through the cancer thing. She can give her some helpful advice, I'm sure."

"Uh … I'm not sure Mallory's up for the whole Girlfriend Posse treatment. She's pretty shy," I caution.

Heather smirks. "You have met Tara. She is one of the founding members. Several years ago, when we first started the Girlfriend Posse, Tara could barely bring herself to leave the house. We can work with shy — just leave it all to us."

"Mallory met Tara the other night after Aidan's charity concert. The two of them seemed to hit it off well, so I have no doubt Tara has already got something planned. I've hung around you guys long enough to know never to stand in the way of the Girlfriend Posse."

Tyler clears his throat. "The guys don't have a fancy name or anything, but we're here for you too. Just let us know if you need anything, okay?"

I point down at the bag from her bakery, Joy and Tiers. "Yeah, I kinda figured. Thanks."

"Well, I've got to go work on a large wedding cake order. But I hope everything goes as well as it can under the circumstances," Heather says as she squeezes my hand one last time.

"Me too." I try to keep from choking up.

"You want more ice chips?" I take a moment to fix the crooked oximeter on Mallory's finger.

Mallory shakes her head. "No, what I really want is food! I'm starving."

"If you keep these down, I bet they'll let you have some soft stuff after the next set of vitals. They want you to take it easy on your stomach for a bit. If you start throwing up, it's tough on your stitches."

Tears leak out of the corners of Mallory's eyes. "I knew this was coming. All the tests pointed in this direction. But somehow, I'm still shocked. I mean, how ridiculous am I? Even Mindy warned me this would happen. How many people have their own personal psychic give them a heads up? Yet here I am still stunned that I'm a B cup on one side and an A-and-a-half on the other."

"I think you're beating yourself up over nothing. It doesn't matter if you were prepared or not, having a cancer diagnosis confirmed is a big deal."

"You know what's bothering me? My breasts weren't pin-up material to begin with, but pretend husband or not, you won't ever get the chance to see me whole. The version of me you'll see will be a damaged, disfigured one."

I grasp Mallory's hand and warm it between mine. "Well, here's something you don't know about me. I've never been a breast or leg kind of guy. I'm more about a woman whose eyes sparkle with glee when she has a fabulous secret or a woman who can spin words like a ninja weapon yet string them together like beautiful poetry. I'm all about a woman whose heart is big enough to cherish a lonely older woman like a family member and respect her friend's unconventional relationship as if it's no big deal. That's what I find sexy in a woman. Do I care about your breasts? Yes — but, only to the extent that I don't want them to kill you."

Mallory's eyes squeeze shut and when she opens them again, she pins me with a serious gaze. "Are you really this perfect or are you merely saying these things to make me feel better?"

"No, I'm not so perfect. You can ask the guys I work with; they'll tell you I have lots of flaws. I am prone to snoring. I can't cook pasta correctly to save my soul — it always turns out raw or too mushy — no matter how many times I try. My handwriting is atrocious. And according to everyone who works at the firehouse, I load the dishwasher incorrectly. Despite it all, I mean exactly what I said —how you look matters little to me."

Through a teary grin, Mallory says, "I guess we'll have to do some negotiations, I take my dishwasher logistics quite seriously."

When I hear a soft knock on the door frame, I spin around in surprise. The woman laughs at my ferocious expression. "Relax, I know I look a little tired, but I believe we've met before. I'm Dr. Callie Stephenson. I operated on your wife today." She reaches out to shake my hand.

When she reaches Mallory's bedside, she briefly checks her chart and her vitals. "I'm sorry we had to find any cancer at all, but the areas we did find seemed well contained. There is some concern regarding the pathology of your lymph node. Out of an abundance of caution, I'd like you to have a couple of short courses of chemotherapy. Your margins look clean."

Mallory slumps deeper into the bed. "I was doing a little research — it's kind of what I do. Chemotherapy means I might not have kids."

The doctor nods. "It's true, chemotherapy can negatively affect fertility. You are relatively young and I don't anticipate more than a few weeks of treatment. Hopefully, those factors will work in your favor. If you'd like, I can send you to a fertility specialist and they can talk to you about options for retrieving your eggs before we pursue chemotherapy."

The doctor looks at me. "That would be entirely Mallory's decision. I support her either way," I answer awkwardly.

Mallory shrugs. "I have mixed emotions. I'm adopted and I've always dreamed of having a child who resembles me. But then again, as an adoptee, I understand what it means to have a family who loves you and takes you in. I guess I'll take my chances. If I'm meant to have a child naturally, it'll happen. If not, adoption works for me."

Dr. Stephenson nods. "That sounds like a healthy approach. In this case, it's probably ideal. New studies have shown starting chemotherapy earlier rather than later is more beneficial to long-term outcomes."

"That's the kind of news I like to hear." I squeeze Mallory's hand for reassurance.

Dr. Stephenson goes to the other side of the bed and examines Mallory's bandages and the drainage tube under her arm. "Everything looks great here. Your surgery went a little longer than I expected. You could reasonably spend the night in the hospital or go home if you feel more comfortable. I'm a little reluctant to send you home unless you have great help there because I don't want you to overdo it."

Mallory perks up. "Oh please, can I go home? I'm not comfortable here. I promise I will follow all the directions."

The doctor backs up and studies Mallory carefully.

"Who is planning to stay with you tonight?"

"Would a paramedic work?"

The doctor looks a little surprised. "Yes, of course."

Mallory holds up our joined hands. "Turns out this guy fits the bill perfectly. I promise to be good and not kick him out of the house if you let me go home," she says with big, pleading puppy dog eyes.

"I only wish all of my patients had such great postoperative care. Okay, I will print out my orders. If you have any questions about the postoperative instructions, please let me know. There is a number to call. I happen to be the physician on call tonight so you will be talking to me if you have a question. Come back in five days and if things look good, I will remove the drain. There should be an appointment already made on the discharge papers."

Before Dr. Stephenson leaves the room, I shake her hand. "Thank you for helping to save Mallory's life. I can't imagine my life without her in it."

• • •

Mallory sinks back into the pillows I propped up against her headboard. "Geez, I'm so sorry. I did not mean to puke all over your car."

"Seriously, don't worry about it. Pain medication and motion can do that, especially post-op. Do you have any idea how many times I clean up biological gunk on any given day? I don't even notice it anymore, honestly. I would have been more surprised if you hadn't tossed your cookies."

"Does this mean I don't get to eat? I'm still starving."

"Don't worry, I'll feed you. You need food in your stomach when you're taking pain medication. However, it does mean you're going to start with some chicken and rice soup instead of a double cheeseburger with fries."

Mallory grimaces. "I don't think I have any of that stuff around. It sounds too healthy to be anything I have in my pantry."

"I don't think you quite understand the world you've entered. You remember telling my friends what you were planning to do this week?"

"Yeah, why would that matter?"

"I think I've already told you Jaxson is one of my best friends. But, you might've guessed when we went to the concert, there's a whole group of us who are tight. I was recently adopted into the group when I started hanging out with Jaxson. It started out with a pickup game of basketball, now I seem to have adopted a whole family of friends. Anyway, a bunch of them all cook like they're related to Betty Crocker. Gwendolyn, Donda's mom, is a lung cancer survivor, and she took it upon herself to make sure you had everything you could possibly need to eat."

"Oh no! Your mom told me at the barbecue that she'd make sure I had food too and you heard Edna this morning. By the time this is all said and done, I won't be able to fit in my car — you'll have to roll me down the street like a beach ball."

"Calories are good for you while you are healing. Besides, I saw your freezer in the garage. You can put it to good use."

Just then, Mallory's stomach lets out a large growl. She winces in pain as she instinctively puts her arm over her stomach.

"I'll go get you an ice pack and then I'll work on getting you some soup and crackers. Do you want some ginger ale?"

She nods. "That would be nice."

"Mallory, if you need something, please ask. I am at your beck and call. You better take advantage of me while I'm here. I don't spoil everyone I meet," I add with a wink.

<hr>

By the time I come back with the soup, crackers and ginger ale, Mallory is sound asleep. I gently stroke her shoulder until she wakes up. "Mal, I'm sorry to do this to you but you need to eat."

"So tired."

"I know. I'll let you go back to sleep after you eat, but I can't let you get behind on your pain medication." I try to help her get propped up against her pillows again. I cringe every time she winces in pain. I know it's part of the process, but it doesn't make it any easier to watch. She tries to pull her sweatshirt over her head, and yelps in pain as she lifts her arms up. "Wait! Let me help you, please," I instruct as I set the tray down on the nightstand and carefully unzip the sweatshirt. I try to jostle her as little as possible as I slide her arms out of the bulky garment.

Tears are sliding down her face. "I'm sorry Mallory. Did I hurt you?" I ask anxiously.

"Look at me! I'm a mess! I can't even eat or get dressed by myself."

She struggles to find a more comfortable position. After she settles down, I wipe her tears away with a Kleenex. "I wish you would cut yourself some slack. The only reason you're not in the hospital is because your pretend husband is a paramedic. Otherwise, you would be having help with everything. Honestly, I'm afraid maybe we've pushed you a little too far too fast."

I place the tray in front of her. "I can help you eat, if you'd like."

"No, I've got it. I'm just having a mini meltdown. I guess my new reality is starting to sink in. Rocco, I've got cancer. Cancer. You know, the thing people do telethons for. C-A-N-C-E-R! What did I ever do to deserve this?"

"Nothing. You did absolutely nothing. No one deserves to get cancer."

Mallory takes a couple small bites of soup. She flinches in pain as she swallows. "I didn't expect it to hurt."

"That's just from the tracheal tube. The soreness will go away in a couple of days."

"Rocco, what if I made the wrong decisions? What if I should have done a double mastectomy in case all of this is much worse than it seems? I don't want to have to face all of this again."

"Dr. Stephenson came highly recommended. She is a surgeon who specializes in treating breast cancer. If she thought your choices were ill-advised, she would've said something."

"There's so much information to absorb. How do I know if I've made the right choice?"

"We never know for sure. Medicine is a balance of science and art. We make our best guesses based on what we know. But it's never perfect."

Mallory shoots me a sour look. "Really? That's the best you've got. I thought you were supposed to be making me feel better?"

I shrug. "One of the things my patients like best about me is that I'm honest — even when it's tough news. I could lie to you, but in the end, it wouldn't make you feel good or trust me. So, I'd rather tell you the truth. I wish I had some magical wand which could make this all go away or make sense. Unfortunately I don't. The best we can do is face the cancer and its obstacles one day at a time with the best information we've got."

"You don't think I made some horrible mistake by taking the conservative approach?"

"Based on the test results I've seen and what Dr. Stephenson told me? I think you made a perfectly sound medical decision."

"Please tell me this gets better and I won't second-guess this decision for the rest of my life," Mallory pleads as she pushes the food away.

"I think it gets easier the longer a patient is cancer free. But I've never met a cancer survivor who doesn't spend at least some of their time looking over their shoulder and praying they stay in remission. It's simply a fact of your life from here on out."

"Oh joy, lucky me."

"I'm sorry Mallory. I'm only trying to be realistic." I tuck a blanket around her as I kiss her on the cheek.

"Are you planning to be a stickler and make me follow the doctor's instructions to the letter?"

"That's my intention, yes. Speaking of that, you need to take some pain medication. I'll go get you some water and something to brush your teeth with."

Mallory rolls her eyes. "Fun times, I can barely wait."

"I'm the definition of fun times. Wait and see what I have in store for you," I brag trying to restore Mallory's trademark twinkle to her eyes. "Look what I added to your movie library," I say as I click some buttons on her remote and bring up a list of movies on her TV.

"What did you do? Buy me every movie Meg Ryan ever made?"

I nod. "Pretty much. I figured you'd have plenty of time to veg out in front of the television since I promised the doctor I would make sure you rest."

Mallory sighs. "Okay, maybe just this once I won't complain about following the doctor's orders."

CHAPTER TWELVE

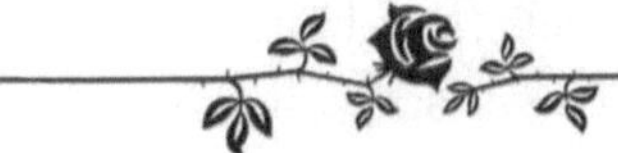

MALLORY

THE LARGE VINYL RECLINER practically swallows me up as I slide into it. Rocco volunteered to take the day off so he could bring me this morning, but I refused as politely as I could. I can't have everyone I know completely rearrange their lives for me. As nearly as I can tell, I'm in this for the long haul. Not everybody can drop everything while I fight cells so small I can't even see them except on slides in the lab. Jaxson's wife Donda dropped me off. She wanted to stay with me — but to me, she's merely someone I play pool with every once in a while, and I'm not ready for her to see me at my worst quite yet. So, I told her I would call her when my session is finished.

A new nurse with platinum blonde hair and sparkling green eyes pulls back the curtain. "Hi, I'm Gemma. How are you today? I'll be your primary nurse during your courses of chemotherapy. If you have any questions, don't hesitate to ask," she says with a wide toothy grin.

I stare at her blankly for a few moments. "The person who put in my PICC line yesterday wasn't so perky. Don't you think it's weird you're so happy? You'll be injecting poison into my body."

Gemma's brows furrow. "I guess it is a little strange if you think about it, but it's not like I'm randomly injecting you with weed killer or something. This is good poison, I suppose. It will kill off the cells which are killing you."

"Yeah, the bad cells, my hair, my eggs and virtually everything else," I answer sarcastically.

"I'm sorry about that. We'll try to make it as easy on you as we can. Are you ready to get started?" Gemma checks my wristband. "Can you tell me your name?"

"My name is Nariko Yoshida, but I go by Mallory Yoshida."

"Very good. Please look at your bracelet and see if we have it spelled correctly."

I wince when I see the white bracelet around my wrist with the barcode on it. You would think I would get used to it by now. Every time I go in for a test or procedure at the hospital I have to wear one, but it makes me feel like a lab animal undergoing some weird scientific experiment. I glance at it quickly and nod. "Yes, it's correct."

Gemma scans my bracelet and looks around. "Are you here by yourself today? This will take a while."

I pat my computer bag beside me. "Oh, I know. I've been warned. I brought work to do. I gave everyone the day off from their babysitting duties. Someone will be by later to pick me up. I figured they didn't need to watch my medicine drip in."

"After I get everything started, I'll introduce you to some of the regulars. Talking with folks might help pass the time. The first thing I'm going to give you is a cocktail of anti-nausea medication. This might make you a little sleepy, but you'll thank me for it later. I see your oncologist has ordered a combination of chemotherapy medications. One I have to give you inter-muscular, or as we call it IM, but the other will go through your PICC line."

"Will I be instantly sick? Under the best of circumstances, I have a touchy stomach. I can't ride the rides at the fair — even the kiddie ones."

"The Zofran and other nausea meds should help with that, but most people have at least some reaction to the chemo meds. If one doesn't work out, there are other options."

Gemma points to another machine beside me. I recognize it from when Andre had knee surgery. "Oh, that's a Kodiak. Why would I need an ice therapy machine?"

"There is anecdotal evidence that keeping your head cool during chemotherapy helps prevent hair loss. There's a specially designed attachment which works as a cap. You can use it if you'd like."

I shrug. "I might as well. I have a feeling I won't be one of those cute bald people."

"Just remember to take it off every few minutes and give your scalp a rest. We don't want you to get frostbite."

"Lord knows I wouldn't want that. What would I do if I had one more thing wrong with me?"

Gemma giggles as if I said the funniest thing ever. She wipes the port under my collarbone with some alcohol. "This won't hurt but you might have a funny taste in your mouth."

"My friend, Gwendolyn, who had lung cancer, told

me she lost interest in food when she went through chemo. I hope that's not so because my friends have made me enough food to last through the next century."

"Everybody reacts a little differently, but some people do find it difficult to eat."

"My friend Andre says he has that all taken care of. He's already bought me some weed."

Gemma finishes injecting several vials of medication into my port. She holds her hands up. "Hey look, no judgment here. Everybody's got to do what they gotta do, but run it by your team of doctors first. Some medications have interactions, including cannabis."

I look up at all the tubes hanging from the IV into my port. I'm suddenly feeling very claustrophobic. "I've got a dumb question. What if I have to go to the bathroom?"

From the other side of the curtain, a voice asks, "Do you mind if I take this one? We haven't had a rookie in a while."

"I suppose. But be gentle. Today is her first day. Remember what it was like when you first started?"

The curtain pulls back and I'm face-to-face with a young woman who looks to be a little younger than me, but she is completely bald and her left leg is amputated clear up to her hip. She waves at me. When she smiles, there is something vaguely familiar about her. "Hi, I'm Sheila. I have chondrosarcoma." At my confused look, she elaborates. "It's a form of bone cancer. It affects the cartilage around your bones."

I must have involuntarily given her the same look people have been giving me since my diagnosis. She chuckles. "It is what it is. I'm here because my family wants me to fight it. But my doctors are a little more realistic. The chances of surviving it are pretty slim. It was way advanced by the time the doctors figured it out — so, basically I'm only doing radiation and chemo to make everyone else happy."

"Wow, that's a lot," I don't know what else to say.

"Sadly, it's not the first time I've done something for my parents I probably shouldn't have," she mutters. Raising her voice, she asks, "So, what are you in here for?"

At first, her blunt question takes my breath away. It takes me a moment to compose myself as I realize this is the first time I've actually had to utter these words out loud to a perfect stranger. Everyone else I've told has been a close friend or relative — unless you count Rocco. In my mind, he doesn't count because he's the one who first told me.

In as steady of a voice as I can muster, I answer, "I have invasive ductal carcinoma."

"What stage?" Sheila asks.

"1B" I stammer.

"You're lucky. I'm Stage IV. I'm probably not getting out of here alive. Mine has metastasized into my pubic bone and it's pretty much inoperable. It's only a matter of time."

Gemma clears her throat. "I think you were planning to answer some basic questions to make life easier around here for Mallory," she redirects.

"Oh yeah. If you have to take care of business, your IV pole is on wheels; there are a couple of bathrooms over there on the wall that's painted that beautiful cheery yellow color. They like us to stay in this room so they can monitor us all in case somebody feels dizzy or something.

Speaking of that, if you don't feel well while you're in the bathroom, there is a light attached to a string you can pull and it will summon a nurse. For Pete's sake, if you have a problem, yell for somebody. There's enough of us out here we can get somebody far quicker than the alarm system."

"Okay, I'll remember." I try to cover my nervous grin. Gemma looks like she's regretting her decision to let Sheila give me the scoop.

"I heard you tell Gemma you're planning to get a little work done. Don't be surprised if your brain feels a little spacey and you don't feel like doing much. Most of us just shoot the breeze or play games. We try to bring a bunch of gossip magazines or watch bad reality TV — nothing too serious. We have an ongoing game of Monopoly. But nobody actually keeps score. We basically do it to pass the time. We sorta have an unwritten rule. You can be brutally honest here about how things are really going and we won't say anything to anybody. This is like a confessional. You don't have to try to be strong here — we all know what it's like."

"You mean like my boyfriend," I pause and correct myself, "'husband' having an apoplexy every time I sneeze? It's crazy! I had allergies like forever before I was diagnosed with breast cancer. Sneezing does not mean I'll die tomorrow. He acts like it's the end of the world when I sneeze. I mean I love that he likes to take care of me, but it's driving me nuts!"

Sheila laughs out loud. "Yeah! Our confessional is exactly for stuff like that. It's perfect for those times when you don't want to be critical of the people who care about you but it's driving you bat-flip crazy. You can feel free to vent here ... totally guilt free."

Gemma chuckles. "I can see the two of you have a lot in common. I've got to go check on some more patients. Your call light is attached to your chair. If you need anything — and I mean anything — just buzz me."

"Is it all right if I eat in here?" I ask. "I was too nervous to eat this morning. I'm sure I'll get hungry before the day is over."

Gemma grins at me. "Of course, you can eat anything you want to. If you're hungry for lunch, I can order something from the cafeteria."

"Words to the wise — don't bring your favorite foods. It's like a Pavlovian dog thing. You'll start to associate your favorite foods with throwing up. It gets ugly. Just don't do it. I learned the hard way. I can't even stand to eat anything with chocolate or coffee anymore and they used to be my favorite foods."

"Wow, I didn't even think about that. I thought eating my favorite foods would encourage me to eat."

"It does in the beginning until you throw them up over, and over, and over again. It's best to stick with the foods you'd eat when you have the flu."

A voice from across the room shouts, "Ms. Taylor, are you planning to play with us today or not?"

The blood drains out of my face and my hands tremble as the information in my brain clicks.

"Whoa! I've seen a lot of newbies come through here, but I've never seen the effects of chemo hit quite so fast. Do you want me to call a nurse?" Sheila asks with concern.

For several moments, I'm silent as I try to figure out what to disclose. "No, I'm fine. It's just that when you figure out who I am, you may not want to talk to me."

"Why is that? Did you suddenly turn into my own personal boogie monster? I'm facing metastatic bone cancer. My PET scan lights up like a kaleidoscope. It doesn't get much worse."

I boot up my computer and pull up my profile on Word Soup's website. "I've been trying to get a hold of you for several weeks," I admit awkwardly.

"You have?" Sheila asks.

I nod.

"Even though I'm an adult, my family still hasn't gotten a clue that I'm not a kid. They still filter my email. Their excuse these days is that I'm too sick to deal with reality. The only problem is, they never wanted me to deal with reality. I guess I don't understand why you would be trying to talk to me?"

I lower my voice so I'm speaking barely above a whisper. "I'm not sure you want me to discuss it here."

Sheila shrugs. "I don't have any secrets left from these people. Almost everyone has accepted the fact that I will die sooner rather than later. The only people who haven't are members of my own family. I'm kind of an open book these days."

I swallow hard. "You might change your mind after I more fully introduce myself. My name is Mallory Yoshida. I'm a crime reporter for *Word Soup, PNW*."

"That's nice. I hope they hold your job while you recover from cancer. I gave up my job. There was no way I could do everything."

"What were you doing?" I blurt as my reporter instincts take over.

"I was working with at-risk high school students

trying to keep them from dropping out of high school."

"That sounds like a great job."

"It was. I hated to give it up — but I just got too weak to go to work every day."

"I'm so sorry to hear that. Fortunately, my job is allowing me to take an indefinite leave of absence until I'm well enough to work again. But, the reason you should care about my job and the reason I was reaching out to you is because we are investigating the conviction of Marshall Todd."

Sheila shrinks before my eyes and she drops her head into her hands. I watch her shoulders shake as she weeps. Finally, she looks up at me. "Marshall Todd is the reason I have cancer."

I draw in a deep breath and my eyes feel as if they are going to pop out of my head. "Pardon me?" I gasp.

"I can't talk today, but I'll talk to you next week — as long as you promise not to tell anyone until I'm done, promise?"

"I promise," I vow.

CHAPTER THIRTEEN

ROCCO

I TRY TO TAMP down my panic. I am a paramedic for Pete's sake. I know all about emesis. I've been trained to handle it, but I've never seen anything like this. Mallory is practically passed out in my arms as I take a washcloth and gently wipe her face. The washcloth is yellow from bile stains. She has been unable to keep anything down.

"Mallory, I need to run you into the doctor. This is an abnormal amount of nausea. It's dangerous."

"Need to take a shower," she mumbles.

"Okay, I'll shower with you. It's not safe for you to shower by yourself right now. You are too unsteady."

"Somehow, I thought it would be way more romantic," she responds weakly.

"Someday it will be, just not today."

I strip her down and place her gently on the shower bench we purchased for her deep claw tub. I put some cherry blossom scented shower gel on a pad and wash her delicate skin carefully. The chemotherapy seems to have made her skin extra sensitive to touch. Last night she was complaining her sheets were rubbing against her skin and felt like sandpaper. I wash her hair twice because she got vomit on it the last time she threw up.

After I finish, I wrap her in a couple warm plush towels and place her under a warming light in the bathroom while I grab a sweatshirt and pair of sweatpants.

"Why am I so tired? All I've been doing is sleeping."

"Dr. Blumenauer will tell us more, but you've been throwing up a lot — that's exceptionally hard on your body."

"My oncologist is a nice guy, isn't he?" Mallory mutters. "It's funny. When this first started, I thought I would only have one doctor. I didn't know there would be so many. There is Dr. Stephenson who did my surgery and then there's the plastic surgeon and Dr. Blumenauer for the chemotherapy. It's a lot," she says as her eyes drift shut and her head lolls against my body.

Her docile posture as I dress her is as alarming as anything I've faced in the last twenty-four hours. Mallory is fiercely independent above all else. If she was more alert, she would be horrified by her behavior. I finish dressing her as quickly as I can and carry her out to my car.

Using my connections at the hospital, I call ahead and give a heads up to her doctor. She needs some fluids ASAP.

I meet Dr. Blumenauer's nurse, Leanne, at the back entrance. I recite the vitals I took at the house and Leanne quickly takes another set after I deposit Mallory on a gurney. She takes Mallory's blood pressure and then takes it again. She looks at me with surprise. "I see what you mean. I'll hang a bag of dextrose and saline. She hasn't been able to keep anything down?"

I shake my head. "Not since a couple hours after she got home from chemo. I tried alternating frozen Gatorade and ice chips. Nothing worked."

"She took her Zofran?"

"She had some in her I.V. before her chemo treatment and then I gave a dose orally at bedtime, but it came back up."

"Let's get her situated in a room and under some warming blankets. Dr. Blumenauer will look her over. He may want to admit her overnight for observation."

Just then Mallory stirs and moans, "Not again —"

I recognize the desperate tone in her voice and grab a blue disposable bag from a dispenser on the wall. I help her roll over to her side and hold the bag up to her mouth as she tries to throw up again. Heaves wrack her body, but only bile comes up. When she's finished, Mallory collapses against the gurney in exhaustion.

"Maybe I was wrong," she whispers. "Maybe I should have just let the cancer take its course. It couldn't be worse than this."

I lean over and brush the hair off her face. "Yeah, babe cancer is worse. I know it doesn't feel like it right now, but it really is. I've been on rescues where we've treated people who are terminally ill with cancer. It's way worse than this."

Leanne nods. "I know it doesn't seem like it, but this is temporary. We will figure out a way to manage your symptoms so it's not this bad every time."

"I hope so. Because right now, I wish I was already

dead."

———◆———

Rubbing the sleep out of my eyes, I trudge downstairs to open the door. When I do, I'm surprised to see Gwendolyn on the other side. She looks equally surprised to see me. "Is Mallory still sleeping? If so, I can come back at a different time," she says as she hands me a large flowering plant.

I yawn before I answer. "No, she's not here. She had a bit of a setback after chemotherapy because she had such excessive vomiting. They readmitted her to treat her dehydration. I expect her home this afternoon though."

"Oh my! I was hoping she wouldn't have the same kind of horrible nausea I had. During my treatments, they told me that they were working on newer, safer chemo meds with fewer side effects. It was my hope she would be the beneficiary of that kind of research. Chemotherapy is the devil. You think you've got it handled, one minute you do, and the next minute you're flat on your back looking up at the ceiling. There is no happy medium. I used to scare Denny to death. I would feel well enough to start dinner with a happy smile on my face and he would turn around and the next thing he knew I'd be sitting on the bathroom floor rocking back and forth like a catatonic person from an insane asylum. I about drove myself and everyone else crazy."

"I'm scared. Mallory is saying things which don't make any sense. It's only been one chemotherapy session and she's already saying she wished she never started them. She wants to simply let nature take its course and if she dies, she dies. I can't believe I'm even hearing that kind of talk come out of her mouth. She was fully researching all of her options before she even officially knew she had cancer. Now, she just wants to cast her fate to the wind? It doesn't make any sense!" I fume.

"Of course it doesn't make any sense! Nothing in her life makes any sense right now. A few weeks ago, she was a healthy young woman with her whole life ahead of her. She had nothing to be scared of and she had the universe by the tail. Now, every time she looks in the mirror, there is a visible reminder that her life can change in an instant and be gone. Mallory only has to breathe deeply or try to raise her arms to be reminded she's not in charge of her destiny. Everything she thought was true about her life, isn't."

"I would've thought at least some of those changes would have been for the positive," I mope.

"Oh, more than likely they are," she says as she squeezes my shoulder. "Don't be too disheartened. But, you have to remember even if you are a ray of sunshine in her otherwise dark world right now; you are all mixed in with the darkness. It'll take her a little while to untangle it all."

I sink down to the edge of Mallory's couch and sit on the arm. "Does that mean our relationship is doomed because of the way we met?" I ask, feeling dejected.

"I didn't say that. It's just a little harder to figure it all out. I fell in love with Denny during the middle of my battle against lung cancer. It felt like we did everything backwards. We did all the tough stuff in the beginning. We faced all the life and death matters first and after the scary stuff was over, we had to go back and figure out how to do normal couple stuff. It was strange."

"I don't know what to think. Mallory didn't even

want me there for the first chemotherapy treatment. She was afraid to bother me at work. She didn't want me to take any more time off than necessary. I told her I would be there for anything she ever needed. *Ever.* I thought I made that clear enough to her. But she didn't want me to go out of my way to help her. Doesn't she understand that I would move heaven and earth for her?"

Gwendolyn chuckles. "I'm sure she understands. You've made that abundantly clear. I saw the two of you together at Aiden's concert. It's clear that your heart has totally made up its mind about your future with Mallory. But, I've been in Mallory's shoes. I know what it's like. When you're sick and you're used to being independent, you don't want to have other people rearrange their whole lives simply to help you. It's a strange battle of keeping your dignity and pride and not wanting to be a burden."

"Usually, Mallory and I can talk about everything, no matter how private or awkward, but she didn't want to tell me anything about her chemotherapy. It was just weird. It's not like her to keep things from me."

"Are you sure? You guys have been dating for only a few months. How do you know how she acts when she's under stress? Maybe it's her usual coping mechanism, and it has nothing to do with you."

"I suppose you're right. In a way, we did things backwards too. We didn't get a chance to know each other very well before things got radically personal and she had to trust me before she actually knew me. Maybe we don't have the proper foundation built yet."

"I've been married three times and I have two children and lots of grandchildren. One of the things I've learned is that there is no right way to do a relationship. I think we all learn as we go along. You guys just have more than the usual number of obstacles to overcome to make it happen."

"Do you have any suggestions? Mallory is going through enough. I don't want to drive this into the ditch any more than I already have."

Gwendolyn reaches up and gently pats my cheek. "Mallory is a very lucky woman that you're already trying to think of ways to make your relationship with her stronger. I wish more couples did that."

For some reason Gwendolyn's remark makes me blush all the way to the roots of my hair.

"Well, I do have one tip. Whenever Denny and I are talking past each other, sometimes it helps us if we write a letter to each other. Sometimes it's easier to spell out your thoughts on a piece of paper than face-to-face. Of course, we always end up talking it out in the end, but sometimes just writing it down first helps."

"That's a cool idea. But, to be honest I can't imagine you and Denny having any problems in your relationship. You two are like the poster children for the ideal American love story."

"We only make it look easy because we work at it. The two of us are both as stubborn as two old mules — and we've got tempers to match. Usually, we try to work on compromises where we both can be right. But, sometimes that's simply not possible and we have to talk it out and come up with a compromise. Occasionally, it even involves yelling. At first, I was petrified. My second husband was the personification of evil. My physical scars are almost all gone now. But the emotional scars linger for both me and Donda. It took me a long time to trust men in general — even Denny. For the most part, I'm over it now — except for the days I'm not. And then I fall apart."

"Wow, it's still tough even this many years later?" I ask, remembering the stories Jaxson told me about his mother-in-law.

"I don't have as many tough times as I had in the beginning, but the bad days are still there. I suspect Mallory will have days like that too. Some days, she will feel like an Amazon warrior where she can take on the world. Other days, she'll be so emotional she'll cry when she trims her toenails. You've got to be able to be there for her with equal passion on both kinds of days. I won't lie. It's incredibly hard on your relationships. In the beginning, I tried to push everyone away, including Denny."

"So, what can I do?"

"First, take care of yourself. Get some rest, feed yourself and try not to get eaten alive with stress when things don't go as you expected. It'll be a roller coaster. Mallory needs to know she can tell you about her worst day without it crushing you."

I reach out and hug Gwendolyn. "I know you came to see Mallory, but I think I may have needed the visit even more than she did."

Gwendolyn reaches into her pocket and takes out a business card and a pen. She writes her phone number down and says, "This is my personal cell phone. Call me anytime you need anything. If you've got questions or you need a shoulder to lean on, I'm here for you."

I start to protest. "I don't want to impose."

Gwendolyn winks at me as she heads out the front

door. "Cancer is a messy business. Impose away. But, remember your reaction. That's just a small fraction of what Mallory feels every time she has to ask someone for a favor. It's not a comfortable feeling, is it? Stop by the Flower Peddl'r on the way to the hospital and I'll put together a little something special for you."

"Thank you so much. I can't tell you how much I appreciate everything you've offered." The door shuts behind Gwendolyn as she leaves. I hear her car leave Mallory's driveway as I lose myself in thought.

Chevy Chase sees my shoelace dangling and makes a dive for it. "Wow, Chevy if it's that hard for me to even think about contacting my friend's mother-in-law when I'm not even shy, I wonder what it would be like for Mallory with her reserved nature."

——◆◆——

When I walk into Mallory's hospital room, she is looking much better. Her eyes are flashing with anger and her color is much better. She is flipping through the television stations with a frustrated expression on her face. I hand her a bouquet of lavender roses as I ask, "What's wrong?"

After Mallory lays the flowers on the bedside table, she flops back against the pillows, and scrubs her eyes with the heels of her hands. "I'm just frustrated. I can't find any decent news on TV and I'm not in any position to write any of my own."

I rummage through the cupboards and take out a spare water pitcher and fill it with water before placing the bouquet of roses in it. "Not a fan of purple, I see?" I remark with a raised eyebrow. "I tried to find cherry blossoms, but the florist was out."

Mallory gasps and covers her face with her hands. "Oh my gosh! I can't believe I was so rude. They're beautiful. I love them."

"Gwendolyn tells me there is a special code to the flowers," I say as I set the flowers down.

Mallory giggles in a free and easy way I haven't heard in several weeks. "Oh trust me. I know all about that secret code. A couple of years ago we had a gung-ho intern who was all about becoming the next Barbara Walters. She was assigned to our entertainment and arts reporter. It was around Valentine's Day and everyone was hassling Winston about being single. He finally assigned it to Candi Sweets — yes, that was her real name. She showed us her driver's license. Anyway, she made it her mission to do the most thorough story ever on the meaning of giving flowers as a romantic gesture. I'll never forget her horror when she found out some flowers have a darker intent."

"That's funny."

"Yeah, it was funny until her poor unsuspecting boyfriend sent her a bouquet of flowers for her birthday which contained yellow carnations and orange lilies. She almost broke up with him for his gaffe."

"I guess those flowers don't mean anything positive?"

Mallory shakes her head. "Nope, according to Candi, they spelled out hate in no uncertain terms."

"Wow! I wonder how many unintentional messages I've sent to people over the years."

Mallory looks at me skeptically over the top of her roses. "Really? Send a lot of flowers do ya?" she teases.

I feel my face heat as I admit, "Mostly to my mom

and my grandma. I hate to burst your bubble, but I'm not much of a Casanova."

"Says the guy who won the kissing contest," she quips.

I grin. Inside, I'm practically throwing down cartwheels. The fact that Mallory can joke with me tells me she's made a complete turnaround from yesterday.

I clear my throat as I try to change the subject. "So, do you approve of the message I sent with my flowers?"

She struggles to lean forward to get the vase off the bedside table. I lift them for her and let her smell them. Unlike most flowers from floral shops, these still smell like the roses from my mother's garden. She breathes in deeply and looks up at me with a beautiful smile. "I never expected to say this. But yes, I approve. I didn't believe in love at first sight until I met you. I wasn't even looking for it. I was a diehard career woman chasing the next story. I thought maybe some hard-hitting news organization might find me. I wasn't looking forward to relocating to one of the big cities like New York, Chicago or LA, but I figured that was the only way to make my mark on the world. As much as I like my job at *Word Soup*, I always figured it was a steppingstone to something bigger. I never expected life to throw me the biggest curve ball ever."

"Am I the curve ball or just a happy side effect?" I ask, only half kidding.

"I'm not sure," Mallory confesses. "At this point, does it really matter? I wouldn't have one without the other."

Dr. Blumenauer peeks his head around the corner. "Good afternoon, Ms. Yoshida. The nurses tell me you are doing much better today. I understand you are voiding appropriately and you've kept down some soup and Jell-O. Your vitals look much better today. Would you like to go home?" When he sees Mallory nod vigorously, he takes out his stethoscope and checks her breathing sounds and her heart rate. After he listens for a few moments, he nods. "Everything sounds great. I'll review your chemotherapy protocol and see if I can find something that's a little less harsh on your system. I'd like you to rest for the rest of today and start chemo again tomorrow. I'll give you more anti-nausea medication. Please try to stay well hydrated. I'd like you to have some cushion in case the next round makes you ill as well."

He turns to me. "I take it you understand how important hydration and nutrition is?"

"I do," I reply, feeling as if he can see all the way into my soul.

He just smiles and shakes my hand. "Good! I love it when the spouses are supportive."

I swallow hard, but say nothing.

"I will issue the discharge orders right now." Dr. Blumenauer reaches into his pocket and hands me a business card. "Call me if you need anything."

My stomach flops over nervously. Something tells me this may not be the only crisis we face during this process. With trembling hands, I take his card and tuck it into the special place in my wallet where I keep lucky lottery tickets and the picture of my friend I lost to Leukemia when I was in elementary school. The idea that Mallory's picture could join his gives me nightmares. Even though all the signs point to a positive outcome, after a night like we just had, it's hard to stay hopeful.

After Dr. Blumenauer leaves the room, I crawl up in bed next to Mallory and cuddle her to my chest. "Did you hear what he said? We finally get to go home. Let me tell you Chevy Chase misses you like crazy. I am no longer his favorite person."

"I told you if you let your cat come visit me, he might never leave. Edna feeds him like he's a celebrity."

The corner of my mouth lifts as I concede, "Edna feeds *everybody* like they're a celebrity."

"I tried to warn you. Why do you think I run the bleachers at the high school? It's not because I like it. It's simply a defense mechanism."

I pat my stomach. "I am beginning to understand why. When you're feeling better, we'll have to run together. I don't want to get so chubby I can't lift gurneys."

Chapter Fourteen

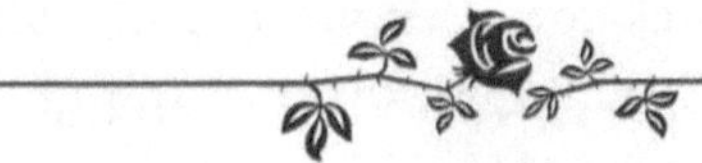

Mallory

I'M SO NERVOUS, MY stomach is in knots. Weirdly enough, it's not because of the chemo. It probably should be, but it's not. I know I'll likely be spending the night hunched over a puke bowl. I resigned myself to the fact that there's nothing I can do about it — it's my life now.

There are a couple of married reporters on our team at Word Soup. In the past, I've heard them talk about how difficult it is to keep confidential stories away from their spouses. I remember rolling my eyes in irritation. As reporters, we keep things confidential all the time. How different could it be? Now I understand how shortsighted I was. For two days, I've been dying to tell Rocco about the development in my story. But I can't — I promised.

I was so anxious to get here this morning; I asked Mindy to drop me off before she went to the studio for rehearsal. Of course, I didn't have to say anything to her. She already knew. As I was getting out of the car, she put her hand on my arm and said, "Remember to judge her choices by the shoes she was wearing, not the ones you would've worn."

For such a young woman, Mindy talks like an old sage from a fairytale book.

I'm trying to leaf through a gossip magazine and look casual when Gemma comes into the treatment room. When she notices me sitting there, she looks startled. "Oh okay… I can't say my patients are usually anxious to come back for a second round." She double checks her watch. "You know you're early, right?"

I nod. "I figured I'd better show up before I lose my nerve, I got pretty sick last time."

"Don't worry, Dr. Blumenauer left us some notes and adjusted your medication. Hopefully, this time won't be quite so rough. Give me a few moments to go get it drawn up. We'll give you a slightly different cocktail of anti-nausea meds. These are a little stronger."

I hold the tabloid magazine up. "Go ahead, take your time. I'm always curious to know what's going on with the royal family."

"Oh, girl — you know you can't believe half the stuff you read. If that stuff were true, William and Kate would have four dozen kids by now."

"Yeah, I know. But I don't usually take the time to read this stuff, so I find it fascinating."

Gemma shrugs. "To each his own."

When Gemma comes back to give me my medication, I summon the nerve to ask her a question. "I know I've been warned that I might not feel up to working. But if I did, is there a private space I might be able to work?"

Gemma bites her lip. "We have a small overflow room we sometimes use for patients who get bad headaches. I suppose you could use it — but, I'd have to kick you out of it if we get a patient who needs it. Is that all right with you?"

"Not a problem — I totally understand."

"You have to promise me you'll use your call light if you start feeling sick."

"I will. What if I interview another patient?"

"Is it about the treatment they receive here? You're not doing an exposé on our medical facility or anything are you?" Gemma asks with wide eyes.

I shake my head vehemently. "No, nothing of the sort. You all have treated me brilliantly here. That's part of the reason I want to pursue this project. It is completely unrelated to my breast cancer. I'm trying to get my life back in order and have a semblance of my normal life. This will help me pass the time and remember the person I was before I got cancer. Who knows, I may not even be strong enough to do it — but I'd like to give it a shot."

Gemma looks uncertain, but then she sighs. "I suppose if you have the releases and all the legal stuff in order from the other patient, it seems like a good idea — maybe the other person will be distracted too."

"Thank you so much for being flexible. We'll try not to get in your way."

"Just remember, if you need anything don't hesitate to ask. The medical staff is here to help you." Gemma says as she wipes off the end of my port and starts to inject medication.

By the time Sheila arrives, I am practically jumping out of my seat with anticipation. I've already done all the mundane tasks I can do on my computer. I've sorted my email, cleaned out my junk mail, and deleted duplicate files. Heck, I've even gone through my pictures and sorted them into logical folders so someday I can print them out into memory books. I sent Andre some funny jokes and even sent my parents a thank-you letter for coming out to be with me during my first surgery.

After a while, I get desperate and take a few weird selfies to send to Rocco. I guess I should've known he would reciprocate and send me his own strange selfies with his partner. I can't wait to meet his partner, Raylene. We've talked over FaceTime several times and she seems like an incredibly fun person.

I am about to jump out of my skin when Sheila taps me on the shoulder and says, "If you're done messing around on your computer, I'm ready to talk."

"Thank you so much. I'm grateful you trust me with your story —"

She holds up her hand to stop me. "Don't start with the mushy stuff or I'll lose my nerve."

"Okay, I arranged a private place to meet."

"Great, I was planning to ask them to put us in the headache room. But I guess you already thought of that. Let me tell Gemma where we'll be. You might want to grab your quilt. It's colder than a polar bear's behind in that room."

"You've been in there before?"

"Yeah, one day Mike was nice enough to hide me out there when my family brought a bunch of people to see me."

"You were hiding from your own family? Wow! I thought I had a rough relationship with my parents."

"You have no idea. I would hide from them every day

of the week if I could. Unfortunately, this stupid cancer has made it so I have to interact with them. If I could, I would move to Alaska."

Gemma sees me gathering up my stuff. "Ready to go into 102A?"

I look over at Sheila. "We are."

Gemma looks alarmed. She pulls the fabric curtain around us before she abruptly asks, "You're going in there with Sheila Taylor?" she whispers.

"I am. Is that a problem?"

"Well, she has a reputation for being … unpredictable," Gemma answers in a breathy voice.

"Wouldn't be the first time I've interviewed someone like that." I murmur from behind my hand. Louder, I say, "Thank you. We'll let you know if we need anything."

Sheila and I march down the hall in weird synchronization while we push our IV poles. She smirks. "I bet you don't always get warned off of your interview subjects."

I smile. "It happens more regularly than you might imagine. My assistant is a bit of a worrywart. He screens nearly everyone I talked to, including my trainer at the gym and the barista down the street."

We sit down in big beige chairs. As I take out my computer and set it up, a video from Rocco pops up. I take a moment to sip on some Gatorade while I watch Rocco and Raylene lip-synch to a Bruno Mars song.

"What does your assistant think of the guy who sends you funny pictures?"

"Remarkably, Andre likes Rocco."

"Are you serious? Those are their names? Do you

realize your life sounds like it came out of central casting from some cheesy 80s soap opera?"

Sheila's comment makes me almost choke on my Gatorade. "You don't even know the half of it. One of the other reporters is named Winston and one of our interns right now is Harmony."

"Oh man, where are the reality cameras when you need them?"

"You haven't heard the best one yet. Our chief financial officer is Drake Edward Andrew Doleman, the Third."

Sheila snorts. "Umm… I'm pretty sure someone has pointed out to him that his initials spell dead."

"Probably every single day of junior high, which might explain his personality. It's dead on," I reply with an unladylike peal of laughter.

"I thought my initials were bad. Since my mom remarried, officially, I'm STD."

"Oh, I didn't know your parents got divorced."

Sheila adjusts her IV tubing. "I might as well tell you this in order, because it's all related."

"Okay, give me a second to get organized." I shut down my computer and pull out a small recorder. "Do you mind if I record this for my own records? I know you mentioned I might get spacey and I don't want to miss anything. If you start to feel bad, we can stop too."

"No, look … I haven't felt like myself for like four years. I'm running out of time. I have to tell somebody the truth — the whole truth. Not the story other people want me to share, not the story my lawyers would like me to say, not the story which might be in my best interest to tell. For once, I want to tell somebody the real, ugly God's honest truth. Who knows, it may be like the preacher said, it may set me free. I might be able to die in peace."

"Okay. I want you to have peace with your decision, whatever happens with your health." I open a file and pull out some paperwork. "First, I have to take care of some legal stuff. You know, my bosses like to know I didn't hold you at gunpoint or trick you into divulging secret information. This is simply an acknowledgment that you are talking to me of your own free will and I did not coerce you into talking to me, nor did I pay you for this information. If you initial here, it means you consent to having our conversation taped."

"Yeah, I looked up your stuff after we talked the other day. You write legit stuff. You're not any junk tabloid reporter." Sheila takes the pen from me and signs it. Then, she initials the form so I can record our conversations.

"Thank you." I put the paperwork back in the file and grab a legal pad to take notes. I set my recorder on the desk and press record.

I state the date and the time. "This is Mallory Yoshida and Sheila Taylor discussing the case of Marshall Todd. This is interview one."

I pause to take a drink of water.

"Let's talk about the very beginning of the story. How did you and Marshall meet?"

"My dad had gotten a new job, and we had to move from Idaho to Oregon. I didn't want to come. I wanted to stay behind with my friends from high school because who wants to switch schools in the middle of their freshman year? I knew I would be instantly unpopular. I

was always a weird kid. I used to like poetry and music —
but I wasn't particularly musical. I was a terrible athlete,
so I didn't fit in with the jocks. I wasn't a girly girl so I
didn't fit in with the chicks, but I wasn't a gamer so I
didn't fit in with those guys either. My parents were so
afraid I was going to get caught up in drugs and alcohol,
they policed my every move. They treated me like I was
in the sixth grade instead of the ninth grade."

"I can relate. My parents were a little overprotective."

"The constant supervision ticked me off. I started
evading them and acting more wild than I actually was. I
hung out with this dude who had pierced ears and tattoos.
I knew he was the kind of guy my dad would hate — but
that was the point, really. It was all fun and games until
Axel backhanded me hard enough to send me into the
lockers."

"Oh wow!"

I definitely saw stars. Afterwards, I puked in the
bushes outside of the school.

"Marshall Todd happened to be walking by while I
was throwing up. He didn't see what happened earlier, so
he assumed I was throwing up because I'd been drinking.
He said, 'You need to take better care of yourself. You're
too smart and pretty to throw your life away like that.'"

"Ouch," I mutter under my breath.

"I got right up in his face and screamed at him that
he had no idea what he was talking about."

"Good for you."

"He just smiled and said, 'I don't know what your
deal is, but most girls around here like it when I throw
them a compliment.' I was so angry — but mostly
embarrassed. Even though he thought I was fall down

drunk, he helped me get cleaned up and safely home. To this day, I have mixed emotions about the encounter. He was having fun at my expense, yet he was still remarkably kind and tender."

"I can imagine."

"A few months later, I started dating one of his teammates. I hid Tyrone from my parents because I wasn't even supposed to be dating. I wasn't sixteen yet. I told my parents I was on yearbook and had to go to all the school events. They were thrilled because they thought it meant I was finally fitting in at a new school — for the first time in my life. I bought a cheap digital camera at Walmart and was showing my family all the pictures I was taking of the athletes and cheerleaders at school — you know, like at pep rallies, basketball games, and the soccer players playing on the field. My parents ate my lies up."

"Impressive amount of deviousness; my teenage self is jealous of your thoroughness."

"In the meantime, I was playing the role of a lifetime with Tyrone. For once in my life, I was a popular kid hanging out with the jock. It was like a dream come true."

"As a former band geek, I can totally relate."

"I thought everything was perfect, but Marshall knew something I didn't know. Apparently, Tyrone had a list of girls he was planning to sleep with during the school year. There was some weird scavenger hunt game in which the guys got points for 'bagging' as many chicks on the list as they possibly could. I was one of many. Unfortunately, I found out in the middle of a party after I had just slept with Tyrone. The more popular girls at the party were taunting me mercilessly."

"How awful for you."

"Oh, you have no idea. Because during this same incident, my parents learned how to turn on the tracking features on my cell phone and decided to track me down and haul me home. Unfortunately for Marshall, he was in the middle of breaking the news about the scavenger hunt and Tyrone's nefarious plans when my dad burst in and caught Marshall giving me a hug and trying to comfort me. They hauled Marshall down to the police station. I wanted to go to the hospital to have a rape kit done, but my dad refused. I knew it would have shown Marshall didn't touch me, but it didn't matter to them when I told them Marshall hadn't done anything to me. Of course, my credibility was immediately called into question after I admitted I'd recently had sex. When they searched my phone, they found the snarky messages I had sent him. I was fifteen, he was eighteen, I was at a party without my parent's permission and I had been drinking. I was powerless."

"That's interesting — the lead which led me to pursue this case said there was no DNA match."

"Technically, that's true. There wasn't one because my parents wouldn't let them take a sample. Without it, I couldn't prove Marshall didn't attack me. Not a single soul was listening to me. No one was on my side. By the time the police were done with me, I was beginning to doubt what happened myself. Honestly, I had been drinking. I never touched any drugs though. I only wanted to fit in. So, I had pineapple juice and vodka. My dad didn't even know — probably still doesn't know to this day — that I got the alcohol from his 'fancy Christmas booze' stash. My parents only drank it between Thanksgiving and New Year's so they always forgot what was in it."

Sheila takes a gulp of water before she continues. "In my heart I knew Marshall Todd didn't do anything to me. I mean, he wasn't my favorite person. I thought he was a little self-righteous and a little too into himself you know, being a jock and all? The way people talked, he was so good at basketball and he had a full ride scholarship lined up from about the time he was in the seventh grade. I don't even know why he was at that party because he was all about taking care of his body. I never saw him drink anything except water or protein shakes. He ate hard-boiled eggs and chicken breasts for lunch."

"Didn't they talk to other people at the party who knew what happened? Why were you the only person who testified at the trial?"

"I don't know! That part never made any sense to me. There were other people at the party besides Tyrone. I guess in the strictest sense of the word Tyrone probably could have been charged with something — maybe. I was only fifteen. I think he was eighteen like Marshall."

Sheila counts on her fingers.

"I dunno. Maybe he was only seventeen. Either way, he didn't rape me like you would think of rape. I consented to our relationship or at least what I thought our relationship was. I was already planning to join him at his university. I was planning to take as many AP classes as I could, so I could skip a year of college and we could graduate close together. I thought Tyrone would be my happily ever after. I didn't know I was only a box he had to check off in a scavenger hunt game."

"I'm sorry. Nobody should be treated that way."

"I tried to tell people I wasn't hurt and no one should

go to trial. Nobody heard me. I said it over and over again. I insisted Marshall Todd didn't touch me."

"What happened? The DA wouldn't even advocate for your side of the story?"

"No, when I got more insistent as the trial got closer, my parents decided my aberrant behavior must be caused by excessive drug and alcohol use and mental illness. So, they had me committed against my will. The 'treatment program' drugged me up so much I barely could remember my name, let alone have a coherent thought. The counselor was big on repressed memories. They tried to convince me my natural dislike of Marshall Todd had less to do with us traveling in different social circles and more to do with my suddenly repressed memories of our time together. They said Marshall was only at the party to pimp me out to Tyrone and that he was truly a bad guy who had to be stopped. They drilled this into my head over and over again. It was almost as if they were lines of a play I needed to rehearse. If I tried to disagree and tell them what really happened, they gave me more drugs and told me I would never get to go home and see my little sister. Finally, I was too weak to fight anymore. I told them what they wanted to hear, just so I could go home and sleep in my own bed, listen to my own music, and write my own poetry. I simply wanted it all to go away."

"I can't say I wouldn't do the same thing, if I were in your shoes."

"You're just saying that. What I did is horrible. I ruined someone's life forever."

"At the time, you couldn't know what would happen," I counter. "I'm sure you thought the police would do their job and get other witnesses to counteract your story."

"I did. I used to watch all those crime shows on TV where DNA is the key to everything, or there's a surprise witness who breaks open the whole case. Instead, the only witness was me."

"Do you want to go on, or do you want a break?"

"I'm good if you are. I want to finish telling you this. I haven't felt this free in forever. Thank you for giving me the opportunity to set the record straight. I thought I'd put this all behind me, but I guess I haven't."

"It seems like you were used for something, I don't know what — but something."

"All these years later, and I've never figured it out either."

"I read the trial transcripts, but I didn't really get a full sense of what happened. Can you tell me?"

"As you can imagine, I didn't want to testify at the trial at all. But, I had a subpoena, so I didn't have a choice. My psychiatrist basically decided I was crazy. That drives me batty. My reputation from his 'diagnosis' follows me to this day. I mean, come on, you saw it today. I don't have a problem with drugs or alcohol — although at this point, I wonder if maybe sometimes my life might be easier if I did. I don't have issues. I never did. I was young and stupid and wanted to fit in with my friends, but I wasn't addicted to anything except wanting to be popular like everybody else. I was stressed and depressed because nobody on the planet would believe me when I told them what happened — but I didn't need to be medicated. Surprise, surprise, nobody listened to me about that either."

Tears are flowing down Sheila's face, but she doesn't stop.

"By the time the trial rolled around, I resembled a breathing mushroom. I struggled to follow the proceedings. I was sleepy and spacey. I just remember Marshall looking at me with this betrayed expression on his face as if he couldn't believe I was doing that to him. I tried to show him I didn't want to be there either. I knew what I was supposed to say. That wasn't the problem. The story had been drilled into my head for months."

Sheila grabs a Kleenex off the bedside table and wipes her eyes.

"One day I tried to go off script and stick to the facts. My dad about had an apoplexy in the gallery. He was making all these strange gyrations as he was pantomiming and trying to whisper the answers to me. I thought the judge might throw him out. I was secretly hoping that would happen. If my parents weren't there, I could tell the jury what really happened. Unfortunately, the judge had great leniency regarding my parents' reactions. The court chalked them up to grief over my alleged trauma at the hands of Marshall Todd. I couldn't believe it! My parents were acting. They were vamping it up for the jury's sympathy. I knew it and so did they. I just wanted to scream the real truth over and over again — but no one would let me talk and tell the whole story. I tried. I tried so hard, but every time I ventured close to the truth my parents would threaten to put me back in the hospital and throw away the key."

A shiver goes up my spine. As strained as my relationship has been with my parents, thank goodness it's never been that bad.

"They said if I didn't do what they told me to do, I could never come home. I knew I'd never get to see my little sister grow up, get married, and have babies. They said no one would ever believe I was sane. They said I was just a pathetic junkie and a whore. I tried to bring it up with my attorney, but he told me to keep my mouth shut and that the real goal was to put Marshall in jail. He told me if I told the truth about what really happened, I could face charges."

"That's basically the definition of extortion! How did everyone get away with that? Your lawyer should have been disbarred and your parents should have been brought up on charges of child abuse, as far as I'm concerned."

"How are they still getting away with it? That's a better question. I don't know if they truly don't understand that Marshall Todd didn't have anything to do with what happened to me, or if there's some larger miscarriage of justice going on. I just know everyone had an agenda and it was far bigger than me."

A random thought pops into my head. "You said your parents are divorced now. Do you think they disagreed about how you were treated back then? Do they agree now?"

"That's the sad thing. It doesn't matter anymore. This whole incident will be the death of us all. Remember how I told you I think Marshall Todd is the reason I have cancer?"

I give her the same startled look I gave her the first time she dropped that little bomb on me.

"No, I don't mean it the way you think!" she responds when she sees my look of disbelief. "I'm not blaming him. It's not his fault. I only mean it like I got cancer because of bad karma. I should have figured out a way to stand up to all the people in my life who were trying to convince me to do the wrong thing. I knew at the time it was awful. So, I figure cancer is the ultimate revenge for my horrible lies."

"What could you have done? You were just a teenager."

"Maybe so. But I was way more familiar with computer technology than my parents. I could have launched a social media campaign on Facebook or Twitter. I could have called news stations — I should've done something. A man is sitting in jail because I stayed silent and let other people be my voice."

I hold up my IV tubing. "I think you're shouldering too much of the responsibility. I don't think cancer works that way. Besides, there were lots of adults in your life who were making horrendous decisions."

Sheila rolls her eyes. "Tell me about it. That's like the story of my life. I told you my parents got a divorce — but that's only the tip of the iceberg. They should have done it a long time before they did. So my mom went from having a control freak for a husband to having a lazy bum who was nothing more than an alcoholic. Oh sure, at first Rodney looked like he would be everything my dad wasn't. He was chill and fun. He took my sister and me camping and skiing. There were no rules. Stella and I could go to movies or stay out all night. We could play our music however loud we wanted or have as many friends over as we wished. Whatever we wanted to do was copacetic with our mom and Rodney. Heck, after the trial my mom didn't give a crap about anything. She had gotten 'nerve pills' from the doctor to help her get through the stress. After she met Rodney, she started drinking all the time. After a while, there wasn't any time during the day or night she wasn't blitzed on meds or booze."

"That must've been awful."

"For Stella's safety, my sister and I moved in with my dad and my new stepmom. It was great for Stella. She and my stepmom, Daphne, got along like two peas in a pod. On the other hand, my dad and I were as volatile as ever. As soon as I could, I moved out on my own. The next thing I heard, my mom OD'd on Xanax and alcohol."

"Wow! I'm so sorry for your loss."

"Don't be. I'm not even sure what I feel. In many ways, my mom was the biggest source of torture in my life. I guess I'm sorry for Stella's sake. She never saw much of that side of my mom. She saw my mom as a silly, funny alcoholic who was the life of the party. She didn't truly get exposed to the dark, manipulative side of Mom. I guess I'm glad she missed it."

"How is your dad coping with Stella now?"

"He is not," Sheila answers bluntly. "My dad put on such a show of being a grieving spouse after my mom died, even though he and my mom had been long divorced, someone from my parents' church stepped up and offered to adopt Stella because my dad was so overcome with grief and unable to cope with the severe demands of parenthood."

I try to keep the smirk off my face as I question her, "What's wrong, Sheila? You sound unconvinced."

"The only thing my dad knew about parenting he learned from watching reruns of *The Brady Bunch* and scary episodes of *To Catch a Predator*. Even before the trial, my parents didn't actually enjoy the experience of being parents. They just liked getting credit for surviving all the trials and tribulations of being our parents. That's why my dad especially liked the theatrics of the trial. There was no reason to take Marshall Todd or anyone else to trial. I was not hurt. Marshall, Tyrone or anyone else didn't do anything to me that I didn't consent to. Yeah, they were a couple years older than me, but it wasn't anything that wasn't typical of a high school romance. I got my heart broken just like every other high school kid. I might've been a little more naïve than some other folks, but I wasn't completely stupid. I knew kids broke up during high school — I just hoped Tyrone and I would beat the odds. We dated for a few weeks and I was ready to send out wedding invitations. I wasn't very realistic, but I wasn't mentally ill either."

"If unrealistic expectations were a sign of mental illness among teenagers, we'd all be in trouble."

"For sure!" Sheila laughs. "But my parents didn't see it that way. By placing me in the mental hospital, my parents got to milk the situation for all it was worth. They could appear as if they were the most long-suffering parents on the whole planet. After all, they had this teenage daughter who'd run amok and was the very picture of sinful indulgence, drinking her way through her freshman year of high school. The ironic thing is that people in the outside world had no idea who really had a drinking problem. That is, until my mom died from her addictions."

I swallow hard as I flip the page on my legal pad. Her words hit a little too close to home. I know what it's like for the world to see one picture of your allegedly perfect family when you know something else is going on behind the scenes.

"Of course, everyone blamed me. I actually heard someone whisper — who am I kidding? They totally meant for me to hear it — that I had driven my mother into an early grave because of my evil ways. A man was in prison and my mother was dead because I didn't follow the ways of the Lord." Sheila has to pause and look away. She turns and grabs another Kleenex from the box as she blots her eyes and blows her nose. "You know, it's funny. When you're a kid, you don't ever believe your life is going to change. You think your family will love you forever, you'll grow up, you'll have kids of your own, and your parents will love your kids too. You never dream that one day someone will announce that you have some deadly disease that's taking over your body one piece at a time and it will someday kill you. What's worse, there's nothing you can do to stop it. You never imagine your mom will die before you and you and your dad will go days without speaking and when you do speak, it is so awkward and bitter, that you almost wish you hadn't bothered."

"I'm sorry it's turned out that way for you. I wish I could give you a special wand to make cancer go away so the world would be a bright shiny place for you again and you would know nothing about cancer and the sad parts of life. If you did have a magic wand, what would be the first thing you would fix?"

"Believe it or not, the first thing I would do is go back and relive the day Marshall Todd saw me throwing up in the bushes. I would tell him Axel was manhandling me and trying to beat me up. I would tell him I was scared to go back to my locker because I was afraid of what Axel might do. I would be honest about why I could barely see straight or sit up that day."

"Really? You think all the bad stuff that happened to you stemmed from that one decision?"

"Yeah, I do. It was the beginning of one big lie."

"So, what if we could start to unravel your lies and go back to the beginning? Would you be willing to help with the process?"

Sheila nods. "Yeah, I thought that's what the purpose of today's whole conversation was. I want to go back and see if I can fix what I did wrong in the past."

"I'm not sure it will be quite so easy. But, let me see what I can do to make this go a little faster." I open the file with the releases and I point to another box on the release. "In order for me to be able to do what I need to do to help Marshall Todd, I need to be able to talk to people about what we discussed today. That means I need to be able to tell them everything. I will do my best to do so in confidence but that might not always be possible. So, I need your permission to discuss what we've talked about freely."

"Well, we've come this far. It doesn't make any sense for me not to allow you to talk to other people involved in this case." She pulls the paper from the stack. "So, how do I do this?"

"See the line for amended permissions? Just sign it there and in a brief phrase tell us why you're changing the level of privacy. Sign and initial it, and I'll do the same."

"I feel like I'm buying a car off the car lot. This is weird."

"It is a little strange, but we don't want anyone to challenge our releases, so we have got to play it by the book."

Sheila takes a moment to read everything before she signs it. "I think I've got everything squared away."

"It is my hope that this will be the beginning of setting everyone free from the injustices of the past."

Sheila crosses her chest in the sign of the cross. "From your lips to God's ears. There may not be very many miracles left for me, but I pray this is one. If anyone deserves it, it's Marshall Todd. He has paid far too high a price for something he never did."

CHAPTER FIFTEEN

ROCCO

I HOLD OUT A new pair of pajamas for Mallory as she comes out of the bathroom wrapped in a towel. She grins at me as she says, "Thank you so much. I didn't expect bathroom valet service."

"You're looking chipper for someone who spent the last hour throwing up."

"I was hoping the change in chemotherapy regimen would make a difference."

"I think it has — a little. You're nauseous, but not like you were the last time. At least this time, you're keeping some fluids down. I think jumping to Edna's homemade chicken noodle soup was a step too far."

Mallory rubs her stomach. "You're probably right. But I was starving."

"I know. We can try again in a few hours, but I think you should go back to ginger ale and popsicles for now."

Mallory looks a little queasy. "I don't know if I can face chicken noodle soup for a while. It's too bad, because I love Edna's homemade noodles. Sheila was right. I should stick to foods I hate. That way when I throw them up, I won't resent them so badly."

"Sounds like a good plan. One order of habanero flavored corn nuts coming up," I tease.

Mallory blanches and sways a little. "You are so mean! Are you trying to make me sick? I just got cleaned up."

"You're right, that was a low blow," I answer with a grin as I try not to let my eyes wander. Even soaking wet with her hair wrapped in a towel, Mallory is beautiful. She shivers so I grab another towel from the linen closet and wrap it around her shoulders as I walk with her back to her room.

She's still having pain when she raises her left arm, so I help her with her pajama top and button it while she clutches the towel around her breasts. The oversized shirt is so long it hits her mid-thigh when she stands. She drops the towel and steps out of it. She balances against my shoulder as she steps into the pajama bottoms and pulls them up. When she's finished, I ask. "So, what happened today to put a smile on your face?"

She grabs a dishpan and an extra hand towel and places it on the bed. She hops into her bed and pats the space beside her.

I climb into bed and Chevy Chase follows, burrowing his way between us. I cover us all with the heavy down comforter. Mallory smiles up at me and cuddles against my chest. She sighs with contentment. "Oh my gosh! I've been waiting for days to tell you this. I'm so relieved I finally can."

My muscles tense as I wait for her news. I can't imagine what she would have to tell me after all we've been through. I hate the thought that she's been keeping secrets from me.

She senses the change in my body posture.

"What do you think I'm going to say?" she asks.

"I don't know. In my line of work, I have to be prepared for anything."

"Relax. This actually doesn't even have anything to do with us. No rescue required; it's actually good news for a change."

I take a deep breath and blow it out as relief courses through my body. She has a point. It seems as if I live in a constant state of terror these days. "By all means, proceed. I could use some good news."

"Remember back when we first met when I asked you if you were contacting me to give me information about Marshall Todd?"

I nod.

"It turns out, I've been meeting with the ultimate insider in the case and she's willing to share her story publicly. This may be enough to get Marshall Todd a new trial."

"Wait a second. There wasn't any real evidence against him, was there?"

"Nope — that's the point. What little there was, is now gone. The witness has completely recanted."

"When have you been working? You're supposed to be resting and giving your body a chance to heal," I chastise.

Mallory blows her bangs out of her face in frustration. "I might have breast cancer, but my brain works just fine. I'm on medical leave, but there's a young man in jail who is wrongly imprisoned. He doesn't give a rat's behind if I'm feeling under the weather. He deserves someone to fight for him."

"But, does that person have to be you? I think you have a more important fight on your hands right now!"

"Look Rocco, I understand you are a caretaker … right down to your DNA. But, that does *not* give you license to tell me how to live my life."

"But —" I protest.

"But nothing! Geez Rocco! I come to you with the biggest break in my entire career — something which could set somebody free from prison and the only thing you can say is you're afraid I'm not acting sick enough for my cancer? Give the care-taking gig a rest for once and simply be my boyfriend! I thought you were proud of what I do."

"I am," I answer defensively. "I'm just worried about you. You shouldn't be under added stress."

Mallory slaps her hand over her mouth and scrambles off the bed. She grabs the dishpan and runs toward the bathroom.

For several minutes, I lay there and listen as Mallory loses the contents of her stomach. I would offer to help — but I know it would not be welcomed. After a while it is quiet and I hear the toilet flush and water running in the sink. The sound of Mallory's electric toothbrush echoes in the quiet house.

Chevy jumps off the bed and follows Mallory down the hall when he hears the bathroom door open. My heart sinks a little when I hear the door to the guest room creak and slam shut.

I blink back tears. Even though I'm only the pretend

husband, the role is starting to feel pretty darn real. The line between fact and fiction disappeared weeks ago for me. This feels like a real fight with real consequences. I wish I could rewrite the script so I could figure out how to win the battle.

Weaving my way through the tables, I try to balance my sticky pecan bun on the top of my coffee cup as I find an out-of-the-way table at Joy and Tiers. Just as I am settling in to read the paper, Denny comes over to talk. Normally, I love talking to him. Today is not one of those days.

"Excuse me if it's none of my business, but is there a reason you're here and my wife took your girlfriend to chemotherapy this morning?" he asks, not pulling any punches.

"Maybe Mallory didn't want me to take her, did you ever think of that?" I answer with far more venom than Denny deserves.

"Oh, Hershey's Bars! Don't tell me you two are having trouble already."

"Excuse me?" I answer.

Denny chuckles. "I forgot you're a newcomer. That's the Ashley way of cussin' without cussin'," he explains. "I used to drive trucks when my daughter Kiera was just a little thing. I couldn't very well use the street slang of the day, so I made up my own language. Most of the guys on the route knew when I had an extra passenger and played along. It just became a habit, even when she was old enough to know the difference. Kiera is a social worker who works with kids. So, she just carried on the tradition. Now, we all talk funny," he adds with a hearty laugh.

"Makes perfect sense. I might have to learn some of those words to use when I'm trying to put in a line in a moving ambulance."

"So, what's going on with you and Mallory?" Denny presses as he leans back in his chair and takes a handkerchief out of the pocket of his red and black plaid flannel shirt and cleans the lenses of his bifocals. His curious gaze is intense but friendly.

I rake my hand through my hair. *Geez, I need a haircut. When was the last time I got one?* "I wish I knew. I don't know, really. We were talking about what happened at her chemotherapy session because she was unusually happy even though she was puking up her guts. All of a sudden, she started talking about her job. She's on leave, so I figured she put her job behind her and just focused on getting well. She doesn't need the stress. When I told her I thought she was doing too much, all hell broke loose. Now, she's not talking to me. She wouldn't even let me give her medication or make her a snack last night. Mallory won't even look at me. She looked right through me this morning when I tried to ask her if she wanted me to take her to chemo."

The corners of Denny's lips twitch. "Overstepped your bounds, did you?"

"I didn't know I had bounds!" I protest. "I was just trying to be helpful. The doctor warned her she'd be fatigued and run short of energy. I just told her she needed to concentrate on getting better. What's so wrong with that?"

Denny doesn't even try to disguise his amusement.

"Son, it's clear Mallory is your first serious gal."

I shrug. It's not like I can really argue.

"Nothing to be ashamed of. It was kinda like that for Tyler too. He floated around life being the life of the party and everybody's nobody serious until he came toe to toe with Heather and everything changed." He gets a faraway look in his eyes as he smiles a misty smile. "I was there that day. It was something to behold. 'Course it took him several years to figure out they were in love, but that's another story."

"How could you tell Mallory is the first woman I've ever been in love with?"

Denny chuckles softly. "Well, it's kinda obvious. If you haven't figured it out, women don't take too kindly to being told what to do under the best of circumstances and they especially hate it when they're sick."

I lean back in my chair and take a long sip of my coffee.

"Is there a handbook or something? The last thing I want to do is make this harder on Mallory. I didn't mean to make her mad. She doesn't need for us to be fighting."

Denny's eyes sparkle with mirth. "Hate to tell you this, but I've been married twice. There is no such thing as an owner's manual. Even if there was, it wouldn't work. No two women are the same."

I frown and rub my temples. "Oh, great. What in the heck am I going to do? If I don't know what I did to offend her, how in the world will I avoid doing it again? It's hard to work out our problems if she won't even look at me."

Denny looks thoughtful. "You have a point. Just a minute, let me go talk to Gidget."

At my blank look, he clarifies. "I mean Heather Colton. Tyler calls her Gidget so often, sometimes her real name slips my mind."

"When I first met Jaxson playing basketball, he warned me you all were an odd bunch. He was right. As much as I've hung out with you guys, you never cease to surprise me."

"Be careful, I might take that as a personal challenge." Denny gets up from the table and walks back into the kitchen. His eyes sparkle with amusement, but I have no doubt the former trucker was a force to be reckoned with in his younger days.

When he reemerges, he has Heather with him. She examines me from head-to-toe as if I'm a distasteful reptile from the zoo.

"Just so you know, this is not something the Girlfriend Posse usually does — but Kiera is one of the founding members. As you know, Jeff is her husband. Donda is Jeff's big sister. Your best friend is married to Donda. You mean a lot to Jaxson, and we take care of our own."

I glance back and forth between Denny and Heather as I try to put her odd statement into some context. Finally, I give up. "What does that even mean?"

"Just be here tomorrow morning. Denny will take Mallory to chemo."

"Okay, thanks, I guess. I've heard legendary things about the Girlfriend Posse. Hopefully you all can help. I screwed up my life pretty well on my own."

"We are quite renowned for fixing messes and making it all better."

My eyes can't find a place to focus in Heather's classic Bel Air car. "This is gorgeous. I've never seen anything like it except on television. Are you sure it doesn't belong in a museum?" I stammer.

"Thanks, I'll be sure to tell Denny you said so. This was one of his projects."

"Wow! Does he do this professionally or something?"

"He probably could — but he doesn't. He does it if he loves you."

"I can tell I'll have to work on getting on Denny's good side. My car is only a generic import. In my heart I drive a classic Camaro, but my wallet disagrees."

Heather laughs out loud. "I hear you. If it weren't for Denny, I don't know what I'd be driving. Hey, does Mallory need any more soup? On the way home, we could stop by the bakery and I could get her some."

I shake my head. "I think Mal is boycotting soup for a while."

"Oh … it's like that, is it? Gwendolyn had trouble too. Can she keep down anything?"

"Right now, if it even looks like soup, she can't handle it. She doesn't do very well with sweet stuff either."

"I'll try some savory quick bread. She might like that."

"Thank you, I'm sure she'll appreciate it."

After we've been driving in silence for several minutes, I finally gather up the courage to ask, "Are you planning to tell me anything about our mission today?"

"You said Mallory is upset with you and you don't understand why, correct?"

I nod. "Yeah, I was just trying to help."

"We're holding a session of the Girlfriend Posse to help you understand how your 'help' was not so helpful."

I sigh and lean back against the seat as I close my eyes. "Oh geez, did Mallory tell you what an idiot I was?"

"No, she didn't have to. That's the default assumption, until proven otherwise," Heather says with a wink.

I clutch my heart dramatically. "That's a little brutal," I complain.

She raises an eyebrow. "If the shoe fits —"

"Touché."

When Heather walks me into the kitchen of the large old farmhouse in the country, I feel like I'm stepping in front of a firing squad even though everyone is sitting around a lovely oak table drinking coffee and eating what looks like scones. Donda looks up at me and hops to her feet. She gives me a warm hug. Then she studies me carefully and kisses me on the cheek. "Breathe, you'll be fine. We are here to help you, not hurt you."

She turns back toward the table. "Most of you already know Rocco Pierce. However, in case you don't, let me introduce him. A few years ago, after Gabriel went away to college, Jaxson brought him home after he went to the park to play basketball. No matter how many times I tell my husband not to bring home strays, he never seems to listen." Donda looks over at me and winks. "In this case, I'm glad he didn't. Jackson and Rocco have become good friends and Kenadee adores him — and not just because he likes all the scariest rides at the fair."

"Tyler has worked a few accident scenes with Rocco and he says he's a talented paramedic," Heather chimes in.

"That's all great," Tara, Aidan O'Brien's wife, comments, "but what did you do to warrant an emergency meeting of the Girlfriend Posse?"

I pull out a kitchen chair and sit down. "That's a great question — I wish I knew. It must be something serious because Mallory can't even stand to look at me at the moment."

Gwendolyn turns to an older lady at the table. "Isobel, this is not your typical lover's quarrel. Mallory just started chemotherapy this week and is having a rough go of it."

"Oh my. Even though it's been decades, I remember it like it was yesterday. I wouldn't go back and repeat those days for anything. It's a wonder William and I survived those days," she reminisces.

"Your cancer was that advanced?" I ask.

"It was advanced enough, but that's not what I'm talking about. My husband William, he's a former Oregon Supreme Court justice now, but back then he was an eager prosecutor. He was a problem solver by nature. He figured he could study my cancer to death. If he could find out enough facts about what was killing me, he could make it go away. He would flat out argue with my doctors. I finally stopped inviting him to my appointments. I purposely wouldn't tell him what was going on because I didn't want him second-guessing every decision I made."

"I'm sure he didn't mean it that way," I blurt.

Isobel smiles at me indulgently. "Oh, I'm sure he didn't either. But, that didn't matter. What mattered was how it made me feel. The cancer had already taken away all of my power. I'd always wanted more than one child and that option was gone. I no longer felt beautiful or desirable, I wasn't even in charge of what went in my body because even if I chose to eat something, there was no guarantee the food would stay in my body — in fact, I could pretty much count on not keeping it down no matter how hard I tried. I lost so much weight I had to be hospitalized because I became too weak to fight off a simple run-of-the-mill cold. Before I had breast cancer, I was a teacher — I was making a difference. Breast cancer took away far more than just my breasts. It changed my relationship with my husband. I lost my autonomy."

"I'm sorry. I don't mean to sound rude, but I don't understand. You're cancer free now, right? When you were done with your treatment, couldn't you just go back to teaching?"

"That was my plan. I thought I could pick up right where I left off. I even had reconstructive surgery so no one could see the hole cancer had left in my life. But, for me that's not the way it turned out. Even though I had successfully beaten cancer and met my five year cancer free milestone, repeated rounds of chemotherapy and radiation had taken their toll. My immune system couldn't seem to bounce back. To this day, decades later, I'm susceptible to every little germ and virus which crosses my path. As you know, that's not a desirable trait in a teacher."

"I didn't even think about ongoing side effects. That

must've been incredibly frustrating."

"It was. Yet, I think even worse was what happened between William and me."

Heather stands up and pours me a cup of coffee. "Rocco, you need to know — we're brutally open and honest in this group. If that's not something you're comfortable with, let us know."

"There's not much I'm squeamish about," I announce, almost boastfully.

Donda raises an eyebrow. "You might want to rethink that. You *know* how blunt I am and sometimes the conversation in this group makes even me blush."

I whistle softly between my teeth. "Wow! I'm not even sure I can imagine a conversation which would make you blush. That ought to be interesting."

"Trust me, it's happened," Donda insists. "Consider yourself forewarned. Are you still on board?"

"Yeah, I need to know the full scoop," I declare bravely, wondering what I've talked myself into.

"I don't know if you've met my William, but he is a driven man. When he makes up his mind about something he wants, he doesn't let anything get in his way. When we met, he was on his way to trial. I was working at the Five-n-Dime. He spilled something on his tie. That day, I was wearing a tie as part of my Halloween costume. I was dressed up like a gangster. He decided he didn't want one of the ties in the store, he wanted my tie."

"That's quite an opening line."

"Yeah, all the time he spent flirting with me made him late for court. He says that's the only time he's ever been late for court in his entire career but it was worth it."

"He wasn't just an excellent jurist, the man had moves." I laugh.

"You have no idea! From that moment on, we were like fireworks on the 4th of July. You couldn't keep us apart. Keep in mind this was back in the day when girls were taught sex was a duty you weren't exactly supposed to enjoy. Bullpucky! We burned up the sheets!"

"Umm … Congratulations?" I stammer. "I'm not exactly sure what I'm supposed to say here."

Heather snorts. "We tried to warn you."

"Even we old people weren't always old," Gwendolyn teases. "I was once a looker too."

Kiera high-fives her mother-in-law. "Who are you kidding? You're still a looker. My dad thinks you're the sexiest thing on the planet."

Isobel looks over at her friend.

"It's true Gwen, he does." She glances back over at me. "Trust me, there's a point to this conversation. Anyway, before I was diagnosed with breast cancer, our sex life was H-O-T, hot. We had no complaints."

Isobel clears her throat and takes a drink of water before she continues, "Then the big C entered our world and changed everything. All of a sudden William forgot he was my lover. He became my caretaker. Even long after my mastectomy and reconstruction scars healed, he acted like he was afraid to touch me for fear I would break. I questioned whether he even found me attractive anymore. After all, I'd lost all the hair on my head and everywhere else. I even lost my eyelashes and eyebrows. I looked like some strange alien. In my mind, there was no way he could find somebody like me attractive anymore.

I became sullen, depressed, and anxious. My anxiety made it difficult for me to leave the house."

The pain in Isabel's expression makes it clear that it feels like it happened yesterday instead of years ago.

"My depression and anxiety made William's protective instincts kick in even more. If I wanted to go out dancing or for a walk, he would openly question whether I was up to it. If I wanted to go to church, he would complain about the germs. If I wanted to go to the grocery store, he would offer to go in my place stating that I would get too tired if I went. Soon, I felt like I was incapable of doing anything on my own."

I hang my head for a moment as I gather my thoughts.

"Okay, I can see that my remarks probably sounded a lot like that. I'll be honest, I came off like a jerk. She was trying to tell me some exciting news and I stomped all over it."

A woman with shoulder length dark hair holds up her coffee cup in a mock salute. "I don't know if you remember me, but I'm Heather's sister, Madison. So, here's my advice: It's pretty simple. Don't be a jerk. Okay, maybe that's a little too simplistic. I've been in your shoes. I've been the one trying to support someone with health issues. It's hard to help without being pushy. Sometimes it helps to ask if they're just venting or if they actually need you to step in and solve something."

Kiera puts her arm on my shoulder. "Madison has a good point. Was Mallory asking for help?"

I blush. "No, in fact she specifically told me it was good news and I didn't have to rush in and rescue anyone."

"You remind me a lot of my husband Jeff. When we first met, he was still in law school. He was earning extra money on the side as a lifeguard. He has EMT training as well. After he found out I have autonomic dysreflexia, he was always on alert in case my health was compromised. I finally had to tell him to stand down because he was stressing me out. We almost broke up because he felt like I wasn't being honest with him when I got an unexpected kidney infection before we got married. He thought I was deliberately keeping my health status a secret from him. We had to work on our trust issues. He had to trust that I would be honest with him and I had to believe that he could handle it if things didn't go well. Eventually, we got to a place where we could reach a compromise — but it took a while."

"Since I've thoroughly blown it with Mallory, how do I earn back her trust?"

Madison says, "You said she has a big development at work, right?"

I nod. "She said it's the biggest in her whole career."

Gwendolyn and Isobel grimace at the same time. "What awful timing," Isobel murmurs. "How long did she say this first round of chemo is supposed to last?"

"She's got one more week and then she has a break for three weeks. Then she has to do another two-week session."

"If I were you, the first thing I would do would be to apologize with the grandest gesture you can. Then spend a lot of time simply listening to her tell the story she was trying to tell you in the first place."

Gwendolyn nods. "I agree. Then — and only then — you can ask her if there's anything she needs you to do to help."

"I can do that. Does anyone have an idea for a grand gesture?"

Madison grins widely. "Actually, I do. She pulls out her phone. Your 'wife' and I had a long conversation after the concert a while back." She shows me some pictures of long-haired lab puppies. "A few months ago, somebody dropped a box of these off out at the horse farm. I don't know what people think happens to animals they drop off out in the country, but we found homes for all of them. This particular puppy, Ladybug, was placed with a Coast Guard pilot and his wife. Ladybug has completed all of her puppy training and was halfway through an intermediate class when the family was deployed somewhere where they can't take pets. They've returned Ladybug to me. These pictures were on my phone when I was showing Mallory pictures of my Arabian horses. She fell head over heels in love with the puppies. I don't know if it's feasible, but your girlfriend would love to have a dog. If you could make it work, that would be the grandest of gestures."

"You've evaluated this dog and there's nothing strange about it. It doesn't eat small kittens or bite your hand off when you feed it?"

"Those are good questions. She just came in last night, but we dog sat Ladybug one weekend. The only strange reaction I saw was to my house slipper. She tried to cuddle with it because apparently she had a toy which resembled it closely. Even so, she didn't try to destroy it; she kept stealing it to take it into her crate."

"I have to go home and check Mallory's backyard and the strength of her fence. I didn't worry about it too much with Chevy Chase because he's mostly an indoor cat," I comment as I try not to get too excited. I know how much Mallory loves dogs. Every time she sees Sugar Ray over at my parents' house, she grins from ear to ear.

"Just let me know, I'll be happy to get Ladybug all spiffed up and ready to go."

Gwendolyn pats my arm. "It sounds like you've got a good plan to make this difficult time as happy as it can be. Do you have any questions for us?"

The compassion in Gwendolyn's voice is enough to do me in. I swallow hard before I ask, "How do I deal with the fear?"

"Whose fear?" Isobel asks. "Yours or hers?"

"I don't know … maybe both? She's afraid I won't love her without both of her breasts being perfect or without her hair. I've tried to tell her over and over again it doesn't matter."

"You can't tell her, Rocco. You have to show her — over and over and over until the end of time," Gwendolyn instructs softly.

"What about my fear? I spend hours on the Internet researching drug protocols, new treatments and trials with the FDA. I lay awake at night hoping to hear her breathe normally. I take her blood pressure and her respirations. I watch to see how her clothes fit to see if she's losing too much weight. Even when she's at chemotherapy, I watch the clock minute by minute with my hand on my phone in case I miss the ring."

"What's the worst that could happen?" Isobel asks gently.

"She could die," I stammer.

"What did her oncologist say about the odds of that

happening with stage 1B breast cancer?"

"He said the odds were incredibly low. Mallory is lucky. She got her mammogram basically on a dare — but because she did it, she was able to catch the cancer very early."

"So, there you go. The person whose job it is to help her fight cancer has given you permission to let go of your fear. I don't think it gets much clearer than that," Isobel says. "If I were in your shoes, I'd do my best to live life like you've got one shot and you want no regrets."

Chapter Sixteen

Mallory

THE LIGHT COMES STREAMING into the room like a welding torch and I have to adjust the towel over my face. When Sheila sees me curled up in a fetal position in the oversized recliner chair, she exclaims, "When Gemma told me you were in the headache room, I figured you wanted to talk. I didn't think you actually had a headache. Do you want me to go away?"

I roll over and adjust the ice pack up behind my neck. "No, please stay. I'm just having a bad day. I think it's probably a stress headache. I didn't sleep very well last night."

"Were you riding the puke train or did Mr. Perfect and Devastatingly Handsome suddenly have an epiphany and figure out you have cancer?"

I snicker at her description of Rocco. But, she's not wrong. "A little of both actually. How did you know?"

"In the beginning, cancer is very dramatic with all sorts of urgent medical appointments and tests. It seems like there's a whirlwind of breaking news and decisions to be made. But, after that's over and you settle into a routine, the numbness wears off. That's when the real deep down, soul-searching fear sets in. It's not 'Am I going to live or die?' fear. It's 'How do I live with cancer?' fear. It's a different kind of fear. It's harder to talk about. People understand the question of whether you'll live or die. They don't understand when you have to figure out whether you have the strength to have dinner with your family or go grocery shopping. They don't understand the bargains we have to strike with ourselves and the people around us over things we never had to negotiate before."

Tears well up in the corners of my eyes. "Rocco doesn't understand. I don't want to focus all of my attention on getting well. If I lose who I am to my breast cancer, it won't matter anyway. I want to keep working. It keeps me sane. If I have to think about what the cancer cells are doing to my body every minute of every day, I'll go crazy. I know Rocco means well. I do. But do you want to know what the crazy man wants me to do? He wants me to meditate on envisioning my good cells conquering the cancer cells. I don't have time for that garbage. I'd rather not think about it at all. I want to think about going back to work and freeing Marshall Todd. That's what makes me feel powerful. My cancer is only a temporary setback."

"You told me your boyfriend is some sort of firefighter, right?"

"He's a paramedic."

"Oh, that's right. Oh Lawdy, he has had some medical training. They can be some of the most annoyingly persistent ones. He's probably gone to some workshop somewhere which taught the principle of positive imagery. There's probably some truth to the concept. I mean think about it. If you watch the nurses give you a shot and you know it's a big needle, it hurts a lot more than if you don't see the needle going in. I would rather have a nurse tell me it'll be a small poke than to have a nurse tell me to brace myself for a huge stick. Every time I've had a nurse tell me it's a large stick, it seems to hurt a lot more."

I wince at the thought of the painful injections.

"Your boyfriend is right. Focusing positive energy toward healing is a powerful tool."

I wrinkle my nose at Sheila. I didn't expect her to side with Rocco.

"Wait. I'm not done yet. You're right too. Cancer can't be your only focus. There are too many hours in the day." She rubs her bald head. "It changes almost everything about you. It's nice to have something, anything to distract you. I wish I still had my job. There are only so many word searches and crossword puzzles I can do. As crazy as it seems, even with YouTube, Netflix and Hulu, I'm starting to see reruns of my reruns."

I rub my tired eyes. "I didn't help matters much last night either. Yeah, I was mad at Rocco for what he said. He was kind of a jerk. But more than anything, I was mad at cancer for putting me in this situation."

"I feel you. There are times I set my crutches in the corner and scream at them."

"I was beyond rude to Rocco. I was so ticked off last night I didn't even look at him. I know that bugged him. I'm not even sure what I'll say to him tonight when I get home."

"I'm not a professional counselor or anything, but it seems like if you start with 'I apologize. I let a situation get out of control because I was angrier at my cancer than I was at you.', it might smooth things over."

I twirl the pen between my fingers. "Wow, you mind if I borrow your copy? At this point it's better than anything I've come up with on my own. It's pretty much a truth bomb."

"These days, it's a special talent of mine. I don't have much time for BS. Feel free to use it. I hope it clears up the air between the two of you. I am going to go play cards with Elmer today. He says I owe him a rematch. He's probably right. You need to get some rest. I have a feeling you might be busy tonight," Sheila says with a wink as she wheels her IV out of the room.

I'm startled awake by the alarm on the pump managing the flow of the medicine in my IV. When I open my eyes, Rocco is standing at the foot of the recliner with a bouquet of yellow roses. There are well over a dozen. I smile at Rocco with tears in my eyes. "Let me guess, fifteen?"

He nods before he walks over and turns off the annoying alarm on the monitor. I guess there are a few real perks in dating someone with medical knowledge. He turns back to me and says, "There is a cream one hidden in here somewhere. Gwendolyn said you would probably understand."

"I do. Thank you so much. They are beautiful. If I'm honest with myself, you are not the only person who jumped to conclusions yesterday. I'm sorry too."

"I need to say this out loud so you understand. The flowers are not enough. I am used to jumping in and making all the decisions. I did a terrible job of listening to you. I'm sorry. I'll do better next time."

Gemma peaks her head in the door. "All done?"

"Yeah, the alarm went off a couple of minutes ago."

Gemma gives Rocco the once over. "Oh... hi! Mallory has told us all about you. It's nice to meet you. I'm Gemma, Mallory's primary nurse. She's so lucky to have you to take such great care of her."

Rocco blushes bright red. "These days, I'm not sure she feels quite so lucky," he deflects.

"That's not true and you know it. I just had a bad night. We're always going to have our ups and downs like every couple." I turn to Gemma. "Can you unhook me? I'd like to go home. My head still hurts."

Gemma pivots back toward Rocco and addresses him, "As you know, the headache could be exacerbated by dehydration. Make sure she gets plenty of fluid. If her nausea is extreme, like it was the first night, make sure you bring her back to the ER. I'm sure they'll hang a bag of fluids."

Rocco nods solemnly. "Don't worry. We're on the same page there."

"Guys I'm fine. Ever since I was a little girl, I've been susceptible to stress headaches if I don't get enough sleep or if I cry. Last night I did both. For once, I'm feeling bad just because of life and not because of the big C word. I simply want to go home and eat some Ben & Jerry's and bury my head in a bucket of ice and cuddle with Chevy Chase while I go to sleep."

Gemma's eyes widen as she looks back and forth between us with a look of worried befuddlement. Rocco laughs out loud when he replays what I said in his head.

"It would probably make more sense if you knew Chevy Chase is my very klutzy cat."

Gemma laughs out loud as she blushes. "Oh, you're right. It makes a lot more sense in that context."

Rocco clears his throat. "I'm not sure I want to know what context you were considering."

"Yeah, you're probably better off not knowing," Gemma responds with a wink.

Gemma finishes removing the tubing from my port and wipes it off with an alcohol prep wipe. She types some information into the computer and pulls up a schedule. "Okay, you are scheduled to come back on Monday. I will see you bright and early."

Rocco picks up my computer bag from the extra chair in the room and hitches it over his shoulder. He puts his arm around my waist and together we leave the hospital as if we've just been out on a date to see the latest blockbuster movie.

After Rocco buckles me into the front seat of his car, he walks around to the driver seat and gets in. He latches his own seatbelt and looks over at me. "Where to? You have a few hours before the nausea hits. Do you want to go anywhere special?"

"I wish I could. But, I'm completely wiped out and the only place I want to be right now is my bed complete with my down comforter and feather pillows."

"Any place where you're in my arms sounds good to me."

━━━●━━━

I adjust my headphones and glance over at Mindy who is

hunched over her iPad wearing headphones of her own. "I'm sorry to bother you. It seems ridiculous to need a babysitter at my age."

Mindy looks up with a slightly confused expression. "Oh, am I bothering you? Sometimes I hum when I write lyrics."

"No, I'm worried about inconveniencing you. Actually, I'm worried about wearing everyone out. Rocco barely sleeps even though he has to work. He felt bad about working last night because the chemo makes me sick and so that's why he called you to come over. I'm not sure why he thinks my friends want to watch me throw up."

"I understand. He's just worried. It's okay, I've been through this with my grandma. She didn't want anyone around her either — but one time, she got so dehydrated she passed out. So, it was a good thing my cousin was with her."

"But you're busy," I argue.

Mindy shrugs. "Sometimes when I'm writing songs, it's better for me to be in a new environment. It gets my creative juices flowing."

I narrow my gaze. "Are you sure you're not just saying that to make me feel better?"

"Nope — you can ask my friends. Sometimes I randomly pop in on them just to chase down a new muse."

"Well, good luck here. Any muse you might find in my house could be quite twisted."

Mindy walks over and looks at my screen. "What are you working on?"

I tap my headphones, which are hanging around my neck. "At the moment I'm cursing myself for all the things I didn't ask, but I'm trying to take notes from the interview I did with the witness while I was at chemotherapy the other day. My follow-up interview skills were almost nonexistent. A rookie journalism student could've probably done better."

"Not to sound dense or anything, but most people I know don't try to combine their job with chemotherapy. I know my grandma said it scrambled her brain a little."

"I don't find the treatments themselves to be so awful — now the nausea which makes me feel like I'm going to throw up my toenails is a little disconcerting. I didn't expect to feel this weak. These days getting up, taking a shower and getting dressed makes me as tired as when I used to run marathons."

"You are still running a marathon. It's just on a cell level now. You are fighting every minute of every day to save your life. It's okay not to feel normal."

"How did you get so smart? You're barely out of high school."

Mindy sighs as she plays with her braids. "Early in my life I had people who taught me all about the worst life has to offer. Then I had people who taught me all about how to triumph despite overwhelming obstacles. Lately, my life has been an object lesson in unconditional love. I'm phenomenally lucky. All of those people, good and bad, have taught me things. As strange as it seems, I wouldn't go back and change anything. The hell I went through made me who I am."

"Wow! That's incredible."

A strange look crosses Mindy's face. "I'll be right

back. Rocco needs my help for a minute."

I look around the house. "Rocco isn't here. I think he got called back in to work or something. He got home from work this morning, took a shower, put on some clean clothes and was out the door again." I chew on the end of my pen for a second as a sobering thought hits me. "Oh my gosh! I hope it's not something with his parents."

"I'll just be a minute. I promise. Hold tight," Mindy says as she pulls off her headphones and runs out the back door. Oddly, she stops and picks up Chevy Chase on her way out.

I stare at the back door for a bit in befuddlement and then put my headphones on and try to continue transcribing my tapes from Sheila.

A few minutes later, there is a huge commotion at the back door and I hear Rocco laughing.

Curious, I run over and open the door. I'm greeted with the sight of Rocco holding a large, brightly colored, oversized gift bag which contains a chocolate lab that is currently enthusiastically licking Rocco's freshly-shaved chin and nose.

"What's going on here?" I giggle at the incongruous sight.

At the sound of my voice, the lab puppy wearing the purple bandanna turns around and tries to jump into my arms.

"Well, I was trying to surprise you this morning, but Ladybug didn't quite understand the rules. She just wants kisses and hugs."

"Ladybug? Like Madison's Ladybug?" I ask as I hug the squirmy puppy close. I can feel her rapid heartbeat and her tail thumping against my arm.

Rocco nods.

"I thought she already had a home. When Madison showed me pictures, I thought she was the cutest puppy ever — but Madison said she already placed her."

"She did, but the family wasn't able to keep her. So, I thought you could use a little puppy love and happiness in your life. If you like her, she's yours."

"Really? I always wanted a dog. But it always seemed like such a family thing to do."

Rocco winks at me. "Well, you're halfway there. You've got a pretend husband who already has a cat. Chevy didn't have any issues with her. He was just curious."

I sigh. "I suppose you're right. The timing is perfect because I'm not spending insane hours at work these days. The reason sucks, but it's true, nonetheless." I stroke Ladybug's impossibly soft ears. "It might be a crazy thing to do, but I want to keep her." I hold the puppy in one arm and reach up to hug Rocco with the other. "Thank you so much for knowing exactly what I needed."

CHAPTER SEVENTEEN

ROCCO

JUST AS I AM about to get in my car after a brutal shift, my phone rings. "This is Rocco," I say as I try to suppress a yawn.

"Hey, Rocco. This is Andre," I hear in a voice barely above a whisper.

"Hey!" I answer. "Why are you whispering?"

"Because I don't want my boss to know I'm ratting her out. It's not going well. Philip and I can run her car home later, but I can't leave right now."

I scrub my hand over my face. "Crap! Mallory was so psyched about going back to the office too. I'll be there as soon as I can."

Ladybug and a quick shower are in order for this situation. I make an emergency order at Joy and Tiers to organize an impromptu picnic.

Less than an hour later, I'm standing in front of her desk at *Word Soup, PNW* with Ladybug standing remarkably calmly beside me at the end of her purple leash. When Mallory looks up at me, I can tell she's been crying. Without preamble, I simply ask, "Would you like to go home?"

Mallory nods mutely as a tear slides down her face. Andre tries to come in and talk to her. She waves him off. Turning to me, she says, "I can't talk to anybody right now."

Andre overhears and rushes to assure her, "Mal, I've got this covered. Don't worry. No one expected you to be back this early anyway."

Mallory nods as she collects her backpack and her water flask. She takes Ladybug's leash and curls herself against my side as we walk through the maze of cubicles. I notice people are avoiding her gaze.

We drive in silence but Ladybug balances on the hump between the two seats and rests her head on Malory's shoulder. When Mallory sees me pull up at the park where we first met, she gives me a tearful smile. "No fair playing the nostalgia card."

"I know this is one of your favorite places. Ladybug might enjoy it too. I brought us some food and a few toys for the puppy," I explain as I hand Mallory an extra heavy coat.

I carry the box Heather packed to a gazebo with picnic tables. I knew about Heather's love of all things retro because I'd ridden in her car, but I didn't expect it to extend to my takeout order from Joy and Tiers.

Mallory gasps when she sees the old-fashioned picnic basket complete with red and white checkered lining. When we open the basket, there are china plates and champagne flutes. I look down at my somewhat threadbare Levi jeans, flannel shirt and black leather jacket. "I'm not sure I am appropriately dressed for my own picnic."

Mallory glances at her white sheath sweater dress and cardigan. "For once, I'm good. This is a phenomenal surprise. You know, the kind they write movies about. I feel like Meg Ryan should be popping around the corner any second now."

I raise an eyebrow. "Really? Who should play me?"

"Well, we've got Ladybug here. We already know Tom Hanks likes dogs because of *Turner and Hooch*. That would work, right?"

"You really do have a thing for eighties movies don't you?"

Mallory drops her head. "I do. All the time I've spent laying on the couch recently hasn't helped."

"I have to confess, I've become a Rom-Com junkie too. If Remy knew, he would never let me live it down."

"What kind of movies do you guys generally watch?"

"Horror movies, with lots of blood, guts and gore," I answer as I set a beautiful red tablecloth out and set the table. "Do you want a chicken salad sandwich or roast beef?" I ask as I hold up the sandwiches.

"From Joy and Tiers? Roast beef. Heather makes amazing horseradish sauce. Did you get the German potato salad too?"

"I did — just for you," I respond holding up the little container. As I dig through the picnic basket, I come across a container I didn't order. I smile as I see the note from Heather. I take the sticky note off and hand it to Mallory.

She gets tearful as she reads it out loud. "I hope you don't mind. I took the liberty of developing a dessert for you. I know it's pink — but I swear it tastes good."

For several minutes, we sit in silence with Ladybug sitting on the picnic bench next to Mallory with her head parked firmly in Mallory's lap. Whoever had this puppy before taught her some serious table manners. She doesn't even try to beg. She lays there quietly as Mallory strokes her ears.

After Mallory finishes her sandwich and eats a few bites of potato salad, she sits back and sips strawberry lemonade from the champagne flutes. "Andre called you, didn't he? I swear that man is a Jewish grandmother hidden in a skinny black guy from Southern California. He worries about me more than my own family."

I inhale quietly and let it out before I carefully ask, "Did he have reason to worry?"

Mallory scrunches up her nose. "Ample, but that's not really the point."

"It isn't?" I ask, trying to follow her reasoning.

"Okay, maybe it's totally the point — but what if I didn't want it to be the point? What if I just wanted to go back to work and have it be a regular, ordinary day?" I can feel the frustration roll off of her in waves.

"I take it that's not what happened?"

"No! It was so stupid. By the time I drove to work, the nerve pain in my hands was so severe, I could hardly hold on to the steering wheel and the bottoms of my feet were stinging." She sticks her foot out from under the picnic table "See? I have perfectly reasonable flats on today. You know what these do to someone like me? I look like a fourth-grader. Even so, my feet feel like they're on fire. It's like I've been wearing my five inch stilettos around for ten hours."

"If it makes any difference, I think you look gorgeous even in your flats."

"Thank you, but I still feel funny. If that wasn't bad enough, when I got to work, they had changed my password. It's like they never expected me to come back. They said it was for security reasons — but I got the message loud and clear."

"What did Andre say?"

"Andre said they did a system-wide security audit and a bunch of people were caught up in it. But, I don't know. Andre seems awfully cozy with the new politics reporter. I feel crushed. I've only been gone a few weeks. I thought Andre would be on my team forever. What if he bails on me?"

"I didn't get the impression Andre is planning to go anywhere. I think you might be reading too much into it. After all, he needs projects to work on while you're gone."

Mallory growls at me. "I hate it when you're all calm and logical when I'm in the middle of having a meltdown."

I make a motion of zipping my lips. "Okay, commencing listening mode."

"It was so hard. You know how I was having trouble concentrating while I was at home? I found it a million times harder at work. I never had trouble screening out the noise of other people around me until now. It's like I've lost the switch in my brain which allows me to filter out extraneous noise. It seems to have vanished. I didn't know how to get it back and I couldn't get anything done today."

"Mallory, today was only your first day back. Maybe it's simply too early to tell."

"Oh gosh, don't remind me," she exclaims. "Some people were happy to see me back. Even so, other people acted like I was personally there to spread the bubonic plague. Other people wanted to tell me their scariest story about breast cancer like my cancer suddenly gave them permission to list everyone in their life they'd lost to the disease. Trust me when I tell you I don't need to hear that stuff right now. I'm barely hanging on by my fingernails. I'm so weak I feel dizzy and lightheaded even when I eat. I am not a poster child for everything going right during chemotherapy. I thought all these symptoms would go away once I was on my treatment hiatus. But a lot of food still makes me nauseous and you know all about the diarrhea. I spent an embarrassingly large amount of time in the bathroom today."

I hand her a napkin so she can wipe her tears.

"I want to be strong, but I'm just not."

"Mallory, you are so strong. You need a different definition of what strong looks like. Strong is not your life as you once knew it. It's coping with all the garbage that's coming your way and doing your best."

"But, I have work to do. Very critical, lifesaving work — a man is in prison who shouldn't be."

"I know. And what you are doing for him is incredible. I'm not asking you to stop. We just need to come up with another plan of attack which will work with where you're at right now. You just had surgery a few weeks ago and your body is being bombarded with poison. It's not a shock that you're not firing on all cylinders right now. What's surprising to me is that you're doing as well as you are."

Mallory stops mid-bite. "I think there was a

compliment hidden in there somewhere."

"There were a couple of compliments in there. There's also a promise that I'll help anyway I can."

"Thank you. Right now, I'd like to put today behind us. I'm too tired to think about it or figure out ways to fix it. I just want to eat what I know is probably a delicious dessert from Heather and then go home and take a really long nap." She points to the elaborate picnic set up and the toys sitting on the edge of the picnic table. "I'm sorry. I know you had much more elaborate plans, but I'm simply not up to them."

I glance over at Ladybug who is sound asleep on Mallory's lap. "The only thing I had planned for today was to help cheer you up. I don't think Ladybug will mind if we don't play in the park today. She seems ecstatic right where she's at. If a nap is what you need, that's what you'll get. My only goal is to make you happy."

Mallory opens up the last container from Heather and takes a big bite. She moans in satisfaction. "Surprisingly, for as rotten as my day started out, I'm well on my way to being happy. Thank you for rescuing me. Tomorrow, I'll send Andre a thank-you note too. He's probably stewing at his desk wondering if he royally screwed up."

———•———

The next morning, when I bring Ladybug back from her walk, I find Mallory sitting in front of her computer with a look of complete consternation on her face.

"What's wrong?" I ask as I walk over and try to rub the knots out of her neck and shoulders.

"At the paper, we hire a court reporting service to do

this. But since I'm officially on leave, I don't have access to it. I'm having trouble working from the raw tapes — I need transcripts. I didn't realize how hard it is to transcribe tapes. I thought Sheila and I were in a relatively quiet room, but some of what we said is hard to understand. I'm incredibly frustrated. I thought this part of the process would go by quickly. But it's taking me forever."

"Do you want me to try? Years of report writing have made me a pretty fast typist."

Mallory throws up her hands. "Okay, I'd appreciate it. I'm not making very fast progress here. I'm going to go take a nice warm shower and see if I can work out some of the permanent knots which have taken up residence in my back. I'll let you start from the beginning. You can double check the work I've done so far. I can't guarantee I've done a very good job. Listening to the tapes makes me sleepy."

I raise my eyebrows in surprise. "It does? I would think the subject matter would keep you wide awake."

"It's not that. Ever since I was a kid, I have always fallen asleep when people read to me. It didn't matter if it was my parents at bedtime or my teacher in the classroom. It's as good as sleeping medication for me."

"I wish you would've told me sooner. It might have helped with the insomnia caused by the chemotherapy."

Mallory shrugs. "To be honest, I never think about it because I hardly ever have anyone reading things back to me."

When Mallory stands to leave, I nuzzle her neck and kiss her on the shoulder. "Okay, you go pamper yourself. Ladybug and I will hold down the fort."

The Letter

When the puppy hears her name, she cocks her head and raises an ear. She was in the middle of trying to give Chevy Chase a bath. I think he is enjoying having her around. For once, he isn't the most klutzy creature in the house. I swear Chevy was laughing at Ladybug the other day when she tripped and fell muzzle first into her water dish.

After I hear the water in the shower start to run, I sit down and open the document Mallory has been working on and start the recording. At first, I'm simply comparing the two. I don't find many mistakes and I'm riveted by the story. I'm almost disappointed when I reach the point where I have to stop being a spectator and transcribe. Mallory's right, it is more difficult to have to take down every word and filter out extraneous noise. Yet the story remains equally infuriating and heartbreaking.

Ladybug paws urgently at my thigh and whines. Finally, I take the headphones off and stretch. I look at the whimsical clock on Mallory's kitchen wall and realize I've been at this for three hours. I stand up and get Ladybug's leash from the back door and take her out. When I finish, I go in search of Mallory. I find her sound asleep curled up under her down comforter with one of Elijah Fischer's novels clutched to her chest. Her glasses are cattywampus on her face. When I reach out to gently remove them, she stirs and wakes up. Groggily, she asks, "How is it going?"

"Pretty well, actually. It's such a complicated story. I understand why you are so dedicated to setting the record straight. I would be too. I am sitting on the edge of my seat. I can't wait to hear the end."

"You don't mind doing this for me?" Mallory confirms.

"No, it's fine. It's very interesting. I want to bop Sheila's parents upside the head, but it's not the first time I've heard a story like that."

"It isn't?" Mallory struggles to sit up.

I encourage her to lie back down. "No, a lot of times we are called to situations where there's obvious abuse, but the parents will encourage their kids to lie — right in front of us. It's enough to make your blood boil, but there's not much you can do. You treat the injuries and report to the authorities. Sometimes I wonder what happens to those kids. Then again, a lot of times I don't have to wonder because I go back to the same places over and over again."

Mallory yawns. "Yeah, sometimes it seems like we repeatedly report on the same stories."

I brush her hair off her cheek and kiss it lightly. "I didn't mean to wake you up. Go back to sleep. I'll try to finish up the recording and fix us some dinner. Do you think you could keep down some meatloaf and mashed potatoes?"

"That sounds great. Anything but soup," she says as a shiver goes up her spine.

"Okay, your wish is my command."

As I quickly whip together some meatloaf and put potatoes on to boil for mashed potatoes, I send my mom a quick text to thank her for helping me learn to be competent in the kitchen. Of course, she sends me a response to ask if I'm feeling okay.

I told her I was fine. I explained I'm just feeling thankful for supportive parents and the small lessons I've learned along the way.

I slide back in the kitchen chair and put the

headphones back on and listen to Sheila's tale of utter abandonment and betrayal. I can't imagine being in her shoes. When I reach the end of the recording, I take a few moments to do some research on chondrosarcoma. After reading the information on several medical sites, I realize Mallory's push to get on top of this story and advocate for Marshall Todd isn't all about him. Mallory is trying to get this resolved so Sheila can make peace with her past before she dies. Based on what I can tell from what Sheila has said about her type of cancer, I don't believe she has very long to live.

The timer goes off on the boiling potatoes and I press save on the transcript. There is so much more I wish I could do. Unfortunately, I can't buy Sheila more time and I can't speed up Mallory's healing process. The only thing I can do is take care of her the best way I know how.

Chapter Eighteen

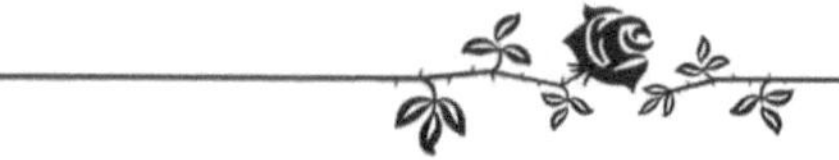

Mallory

I spin in front of the mirror in my sensible business suit and pumps. I look over my shoulder at Rocco. He is tucking in his uniform shirt. "How do I look?" I ask as I nervously bite my lip.

Rocco sets down his belt and walks over to me. Cupping my face, he kisses me deeply. "You look stunning. For so many reasons, I wish I didn't have to work today."

"Do you think I look like a serious reporter? I'm a little worried. There's a lot of hair in the bottom of the shower. Maybe I should've cut it short last week."

"Honey, I look at you every day and I can't tell you've lost any hair. A perfect stranger who's never met you wouldn't know. You look like one of those fancy reporters who cover the news on television. Marshall will be impressed."

The doorbell rings. I put some lipstick on quickly. "I bet that's Tyler. I don't want to keep him waiting."

Rocco kisses me again. "Tyler is a good man. If you

need anything, just ask. He has military experience. He can handle any crisis."

I lean against Rocco's chest. "Stop worrying about me. I don't expect to have any crises. I'm not having active chemotherapy right now. I'm feeling well. I've got a job to do."

"I know you are. Honestly, you've met my family. We are like professional worriers. It's in the genes. I think I'd worry about you even if you were perfectly healthy."

"Yeah, you have a good point. Your mom came over the other day when I was cutting up bananas for fruit salad and she was worried I might hurt myself."

Rocco grins. "See? What did I tell you? I hope you have a great interview with Marshall."

⸺•⸺

Just before I'm ready to go through the security checkpoint at the prison, Tyler lays his hand on my shoulder. "I don't want you to be disappointed. Sometimes it takes more than one visit to build a rapport with the prisoner. Especially one that's been as isolated as Marshall. You might not get a lot out of today's visit."

I swallow hard. "Thank you for the reminder. I tend to get too excited and stake everything on a single interview. I know I shouldn't do that, but I'm really bad about getting my hopes up."

"I could be wrong, but that's just been my experience."

"I hope it goes well. Since I haven't been in the office, I'm not sure if Marshall even got any messages to inform him I was coming."

"If nothing else, it should be interesting," Tyler remarks.

The guard pats me down and makes me dump out my briefcase. When he sees my digital recorder, he takes out the batteries and puts them back in. He does a brief test recording and then plays it back. "Do you have a reason for this recorder?"

"I have cancer and I have developed extreme nerve pain in my fingers. It is difficult for me to hold a pen or pencil and write quickly." I explain. "I use a tape recorder to help me remember the details."

The corrections officer looks at Tyler. "Do you know this woman? Is she telling us the truth?"

Tyler nods. "She is. She is a hundred percent above-board. I would stake my professional reputation on it."

The guard shrugs as he hands me back my belongings. "Okay ma'am, another officer will bring Inmate Todd to the visitor room."

Tyler steps forward. "Listen, Officer Davidson, Ms. Yoshida is fighting cancer, and she's susceptible to illness. Can we use one of the conference rooms instead of the visitor room for her safety?"

The officer consults a sign-in sheet. "I don't see why not. No one is signed up to use it. Can you show her the way?"

Tyler nods. "I'd be happy to."

Tyler places his hand on my forearm as we navigate the halls to a conference room.

By the time we sit down in the sterile conference room, my teeth are chattering from nerves.

"Are you okay?" Tyler asks with a look of concern.

"I'm fine. The enormity of what I'm about to do just hit. What if he doesn't believe me or wants no part of this?"

"Trust me, if he really didn't do this, he will grasp at any opportunity to be free, no matter how slim."

"That's my other concern. What if we do all of this and nobody cares? I've written several stories where Innocent Projects have unearthed evidence pointing to a defendant's innocence, but the courts have said it's simply not enough because there isn't DNA."

Tyler grimaces. "That's true too. But you can't go back and fix what isn't there. You have to work with the facts you've got."

The door opens and a young man enters. He is handcuffed and shackled. He is still handsome, but he lacks the confident air I saw in news coverage when he was younger.

Tyler discreetly shows the guard his sheriff's badge. "The shackles and cuffs are unnecessary. Please remove them."

The guard look startled. "Sir, there is a woman present and you are aware of this inmate's charges —"

I clear my throat. "I am aware of what Mr. Todd was convicted of and I am fully comfortable with you removing his restraints. In fact, I would prefer it."

At the guard's hesitation, Tyler insists, "I can handle it if anything arises."

The guard shrugs. "I guess. It's your funeral."

Marshall Todd simply sighs as he waits for the guard to remove his cuffs and shackles.

The guard looks at Marshall and grouses, "Don't

make me regret this move. It's already been an insanely long day. I don't want to do weeks of paperwork because I was nice."

"No, sir. I understand," Marshall says as he practically stands at attention.

The guard leaves and Marshall appears uncertain.

I stand up and shake his hand. "Hi, I'm Mallory Yoshida. Thank you so much for meeting with me today. This is my friend Tyler. He's here mainly because I am recovering from a round of chemotherapy and don't feel up to driving. In this case, it's also helpful that he is a Sheriff."

Marshall narrows his gaze. "Am I in trouble for something? I haven't done anything, I swear. But then again, that didn't seem to matter the last time."

"We know. Hopefully, we can do something to fix what happened," I answer as I hand him a business card.

"*Word Soup*? Is that some sort of weird tabloid magazine or something?" Marshall demands.

"No, although the name kind of sounds that way. We are a new breed of newspaper. A lot of people don't even get traditional newspapers anymore, so we are based on the web. But we are solid, traditional journalists. We take our jobs very seriously. I cover the crime beat. A few weeks back, we got a lead which indicated the DNA in your case didn't match you. I did some research and found the lead to be viable."

"Yeah ... absolutely... I tried to tell everybody, their cousin, and their dog that I never had sex with Sheila Taylor. But nobody believes a black guy."

"Turns out, nobody believes a teenage white girl either," I remark.

"What do you mean? I was there in the courtroom when Sheila told those jurors I raped her. I got no clue why she would lie. I thought we were friends. I was trying to tell her Tyrone was gamin' her. I didn't want her to humiliate herself. She was throwing herself at him like he was a god or something. Tyrone was a complete man whore, but she couldn't catch a clue. Sheila was new to school, she didn't know any better. She thought he was cute. When he threw her a little attention, she ate it up like it was her favorite kinda candy or something."

"I've spent some time getting to know Sheila Taylor. She regrets what she did."

"Little late for that now, isn't it? All my college scholarships are gone. My mama's life is destroyed. She had a stroke because I was sent here."

"I'm sorry to hear that, son," Tyler says. "The incident happened outside my jurisdiction, but I got my hands on the interrogation tapes. I know that's no consolation, but Sheila tried to tell the truth many times. People stopped listening to her. I don't know if they just discredited her because she was fifteen and had been drinking or if they got tunnel vision and focused on you. I just don't know. But it was a travesty of justice all around."

"Yet, I'm still here. So, what's changed?" Marshall asks defiantly.

"Circumstances have changed in Sheila Taylor's life. She is asserting a little more power. She finally feels like she can come forward and tell the truth."

"Why couldn't she do something before? It's not like I was hard to find," Marshall replies sarcastically.

"There were some unique circumstances. Sheila was

for all intents and purposes being held as an emotional hostage. Her parents threatened to have her committed to a mental health hospital if she didn't cooperate with what they told her to say. She was concerned about her little sister, Stella."

Marshall pounds on the table in front of us. "I told my attorney there was something weird going on. I knew she wouldn't have done that to me. Her dad was doing all this bogus stuff in the audience, but my attorney couldn't be bothered to get up and object. It was so obvious too — like her dad was feeding her lines or something. Sheila looked scared to death. I've seen her face down bullies at school and she didn't look that scared. One day, it looked like she was going to finally tell what really happened and set me free. Then her family created some weird ruckus in the audience. The judge had to call a recess."

"I read a little something about some odd happenings in the gallery in the court transcript. It didn't seem that dramatic in writing," I remark.

"It was all-out chaos. They were even afraid I would escape. I was completely surrounded by bailiffs. After everyone got back from the recess, when they put Sheila back on the stand, it was like somebody had given her zombie pills. She could barely put together a sentence. Everyone acted like nothing had happened and everything was normal. That was the day I knew for sure it didn't matter what happened in the trial, it was over. My fate had been decided. Obviously, the judge didn't care what happened in his courtroom. Everybody seemed to just be going through the motions. After all, what's one more black kid in the juvenile justice system? If one is guilty, we all must be, right?"

"No, not right. Sheila Taylor knew you didn't do

anything to harm her. She never wanted you to go to jail, but she was in a no-win situation: either do what her parents required her to do or lose her little sister. She was hoping other evidence would exonerate you. She was horrified when it did not."

Skepticism is clear on Marshall's face as he asks, "So, why is she coming forward now?"

"First, Sheila's little sister Stella is old enough to move out on her own and not be harmed by her father. That gives Sheila a sense of freedom she didn't have before. Her dad is now missing his biggest weapon," I explain.

"Okay, I might buy that. I would do virtually anything to save my kid brother. What else?"

"With your permission, I'd like to play a snippet of an interview I recently had with Sheila Taylor. Okay with you?"

Marshall looks a little uncertain. "Yeah, I guess so. It'll be really weird. The last time I heard her voice, she was telling the jury I raped her. Even all these years later, I can't believe those words came out of her mouth. I never even said a bad word about her — even when everybody was making fun of the new kid or they were calling her a Ball Bunny for sleeping with Tyrone when she didn't know him. I still can't believe she did me bad."

"Maybe this will help you understand," I reply.

The tape recorder is a little staticky as I ask Sheila, "If you had a chance to talk to Marshall Todd today what would you say?"

Sheila clears her throat. "Well, I know there aren't enough apologies on the planet for what I did. I guess I would volunteer to take his place in jail. That's actually where I belong. Even though I was coerced into not telling the truth, I did lie. That means I'm guilty of perjury. So, I'm guilty of a crime and Marshall Todd is not. How is that for irony? But here is the other thing; I am paying the ultimate penalty for my crime. I am serving the death penalty for falsely testifying against Marshall Todd. I'm at peace with that. I guess it's what I deserve. I'll never be at peace with what I cost Marshall Todd."

Marshall grimaces at the obvious pain in her voice.

"If he ever gets a chance to listen to this, I want him to know I wish I could go back to that day he first tried to help me when Axel hurt me so bad I could barely see. I wish I would've swallowed my pride and accepted his gift of friendship and told him what really happened. I'm sorry I threw that back in your face. I'm sorry I didn't stand up to my parents and scream to the world that you were only trying to be a friend and that you never touched me inappropriately — let alone raped me. I was weak, and I did not know my own strength."

Marshall scrubs a hand down his face and blows out a breath.

"It is so ironic. I did not find out how strong I was until I fought a losing battle with cancer. Chances are when you hear this tape, I might be dead. The only thing I can do to help you now is to tell anybody and everybody what actually happened and the role my parents, the police, and my own attorney played in your conviction. I made some dumb choices when I was a kid. I had no business drinking or having sex with Tyrone — or anyone else. But without a shadow of a doubt, I know you didn't do anything to hurt me. I hope someone listens to me this time. I'm sorry Marshall Todd, you deserved better from me."

I click off the tape recorder. I look around the room and all three of us are wiping away tears. Tyler gets up and grabs a box of Kleenex from a table sitting nearby. He puts it in the center of the table and gives us a moment to collect ourselves.

"What is Sheila talking about? Is she really dying?"

I nod. "Unfortunately, yes. I met her during my chemotherapy treatments. I have breast cancer, but my breast cancer is at a very early stage compared to Sheila's bone cancer. Hers has spread to her pelvis and her lungs. Honestly, she is only doing chemotherapy to make her little sister happy. The doctors have given her a very poor prognosis. It is likely she will die within a few months."

"Why is she worrying about me if she's got all that to deal with?" Marshall asks.

"She knows what happened to you was a miscarriage of justice and she had a large part to play in that. If she can play a role in undoing the wrong, she'd like to — before she dies."

"So, here's the stupid thing," Marshall chokes on his words. "I was totally into Sheila Taylor. She wasn't like the air headed girls who usually tried to date me for status. Sheila didn't even seem to care about my status — in fact, it seemed to annoy her more than anything else. If I got written up in the paper or featured on television, everyone else would be falling all over themselves to get my attention. Not Sheila — she would be royally ticked off. I had a math class with her and she wouldn't even look at me if I'd been featured in the paper or the pep rally mentioned me. It was kind of funny. I started trying to be more low-key just so I wouldn't make her mad. I thought I was making some progress but then the whole incident happened, and my life was flushed down the toilet."

"I'm sorry things turned out this way, they never should have. I'll work as hard as I can to change the outcome. I know I can't make the years you spent in here go away, but maybe I can work on getting your conviction overturned."

"Lady, if you can do that, you're a miracle worker. With all due respect, I had lots of media attention on my case before. Colleges and even pro teams were interested in me before all this crap came down. Some high-profile attorneys said they would help me, but nobody ever did. They only wanted their names in the paper. If that's all this is about, just pass me on by. I don't want to get my family's hopes up again. Like I said, my mama is doing poorly and my dad is working himself crazy trying to support everybody since my mom can't work anymore. I don't want to break their hearts again."

"I know you don't know me very well — but I'm actually very shy. There's a reason I don't work for network news. I'd just as soon stay behind the scenes. A lot of my friends have pushed me to do TV or work in one of the bigger markets like Portland, Chicago, New York or LA where minorities are more prevalent. There aren't very many people who look like me in my neighborhood. I'm okay with that now."

"Doesn't it get awkward? There weren't a lot of minority kids in my high school either. I think that's why I was singled out and charged."

"It's not as hard as an adult. I've had a long time to get used to being the odd one out. I have been different from everyone around me for as long as I can remember. I was adopted by Caucasian parents, so I'm used to being the odd one out — maybe that's why I would just as soon be invisible."

"I know how that feels," Marshall mutters as he squints through the glass at the guard who has been staring at him with a sour look the entire time we've been in here.

I cough lightly to draw his attention. "Anyway, when I was in college, one of my best friends was a victim of crime. I have been seeking justice for people ever since that day. It's like a lifetime calling for me. My parents were not happy with my choice — my dad wanted me to be a doctor or a dentist. It took cancer for us to come back together as a family."

Marshall looks thoughtful. "So, this isn't simply a flash-in-the-pan, stepping-stone-to-a-bigger-job kind of deal for you?"

"No, it's not. Trust me, I've been offered bigger, better positions. But I'm not willing to compromise my values to get them."

Marshall shoots me a tight smile. "I know what you mean. My lawyer keeps telling me that if I just admit to raping Sheila and tell the parole board I'm sorry for what I did, I can get out of here a lot faster. I told him I wouldn't do it because I never touched her — at least not that way. I had my arm around her because I was trying to make her feel better, but I never raped her."

"I know, you know, Tyler knows, Sheila knows. Now, we have to figure out who else knew the truth at the time of your trial."

Tyler nods. "If we can prove the police knew and disregarded the information, or the prosecution withheld information from your defense team, we might be able to get somewhere."

Marshall hangs his head for a moment before he finally looks up at me. "I hope this isn't some weird sick joke you all are playin' on me. I miss my family. My mama should be able to give me a real hug and I should be able to go watch my little brother play basketball and I should be able to show him how to play the game right."

"Well hopefully, if everything goes right, we can bring you closer to that day," I say as I start to gather up my belongings and stick them back in my briefcase.

"Thanks, Miss. I want to thank you for something else too," Marshall says bashfully.

I pause and raise an eyebrow.

"I want to thank you for treating me like a person and not a monster. I've almost forgotten what that's like. I like being treated with respect."

"I'm sorry your sense of respect was stripped away from you. I'll do everything in my power to help get it restored to you. From everything I can tell, it was wrongly taken away."

Marshall reaches out and shakes my hand. "Your belief in me is the best thing to happen to me in years. Let me know if I can do anything to help."

Chapter Nineteen

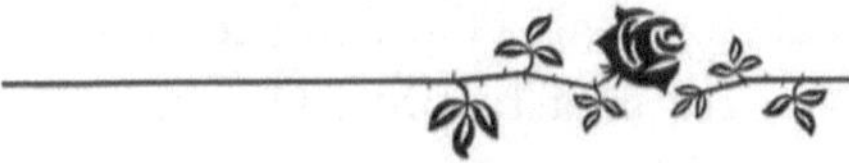

Rocco

As I round the corner with a tray full of crackers, cheese, and lunchmeat for our movie night, I realize Mallory isn't in bed like I expect her to be. After a little searching, I locate her sitting on the shower floor holding clumps of dark black hair in her hands. She is sobbing.

Alarmed, I set the dinner tray on the bathroom counter and scoop Mallory up in my arms. "Are you hurt?" I ask as I wrap her in a large bed sheet and carry her over to the bed.

Mutely, she shakes her head and holds out a fistful of hair.

"Wow! When you do things, you don't do them in a small way," I exclaim when I see a new bald spot on her head. My heart shatters for her. There is no way I can cushion the blow or make this okay.

"I feel so stupid. For some reason I thought this wouldn't happen to me. I wore a crazy ice cap, I massaged my scalp, I took vitamins, and I even used essential oils on my head — some of them really smell funny."

"It wasn't anything you did or didn't do, it's the drugs. Most people who have chemotherapy lose at least part of their hair. A lot of people lose all their hair. That's why it's a well-known side effect."

"I didn't want to lose my hair," she pouts as another clump of hair falls out.

I go to the linen closet, grab a dark colored towel and carefully dry her scalp. It's catastrophic. Her hair simply rubs off on to the navy-blue towel. I don't disguise my sharp intake of breath quick enough. She catches my reaction and asks, "It's bad, isn't it?"

I clear my throat lightly as I debate how to answer. "Well, look on the bright side. You won't be spending a lot of money on shampoo."

She reaches up to touch her scalp. "This is awful. I'm not one of those people who has a perfectly formed scalp. I competed in gymnastics when I was younger. I've probably got dents and scars on my head everywhere."

I climb up on the bed and face her. I grasp her hands between mine. "Mallory look at me. I love you. I don't care if you have hair or breasts. I don't care if you can wear high heels or not. That's all cosmetic stuff and it doesn't matter to me."

Mallory lets out a shuddering sob.

"I love who you are on the inside. I love the person you are. I love that you help your neighbor do things she's scared of. I love that you go over and listen to my mom talk about how she names her rose bushes and you indulge my dad's fish tales as if you've never heard him tell you the story he told you two weeks ago. I love that you are the kind of person to organize a bridal party for your assistant even though he's marrying a guy. I love that you're fighting to get a man you didn't know a few months ago out of jail because in your heart you know he didn't commit the crime he's accused of — but unlike a lot of people you're not doing it for money or for fame, you're doing it because it's the right thing to do. So, do I care if your hair is falling out? Yeah, a bit —"

Mallory stiffens and gives me a withering stare.

I squeeze her hands. "Wait! Hear me out… I care only because it makes you sad to lose your hair and I hate to see you sad."

Mallory sniffles. "I don't think there's much you can do about that. Even though I'm not much of a high maintenance girl, I'll miss my hair."

"I know, but I have some ideas. Do you trust me?" I ask as I scoot off the bed and walk over to a spare dresser in Mallory's room that she's been letting me use while I stay here.

I remove a box I got back when we had some training sessions in Portland. I nervously hand it to her as I hope she understands the sentiment behind it.

She carefully opens it up and unwraps the tissue paper. She lifts out the delicate scarf. "Wow, this is gorgeous. Where did you find a scarf with cherry blossoms on it?"

"I went to Chinatown three or four months back. I can't see cherry blossoms without thinking of you. I thought it would be good for you when you lost your hair. I found a video on YouTube about ways to use a silk scarf as a head cover."

Mallory's jaw goes slack. "You've been planning this surprise for that long? You knew my hair would fall out even though I was taking all the precautions?"

"I knew the chances were high, given the type of chemotherapy you are having. We see a lot of cancer patients in my line of work. I don't see many of them who still have all of their hair. It's just a matter of odds."

"You are so sneaky. I thought you were convinced I wouldn't lose a hair on my head." She holds up the scarf. "Do you mind helping me? It's still hard for me to hold my arms up in the air."

"You might not like the job I do. I'm not as skilled as some of the other guys."

Mallory shrugs. "I'm not worried. I've seen your attention to detail."

My hands tremble as I try to remember the moves I saw in the YouTube video. Finally, I fashion some sort of turban design out of the beautiful silk scarf.

Mallory runs towards the restroom and looks at herself in the mirror over the bathroom sink. "The scarf is beautiful."

I'm thankful I decided to follow her so I could see her reaction. For the first time in a while, she seems to recognize the beautiful woman I see every day. In the blink of an eye, it all goes wrong. Mallory's expression fills with anguish and the light and joy fades from her eyes.

Her knees buckle, and she collapses down onto the toilet as she buries her head in her hands and starts to sob.

"Are you all right? Did I tie it too tight?" I ask as I lean down and run my fingers under the edge of the scarf.

She pulls her head away. "No, it's fine."

Instinctively, I jerk my hand back. Mallory pulls the

scarf off her head and gently folds it. She pushes it into my chest as she stands up and inches her way around me in the small confines of the bathroom. Her obvious attempts to avoid touching me stings more than just a little.

I take a couple minutes to brush my teeth and trim my beard. I know from past experience that Mallory doesn't want me to talk to her when she's extremely upset. Giving her space goes completely against my instincts as a rescuer, but I know it's for the best. When I simply can't wait any longer, I tentatively walk back into her bedroom, uncertain what I will encounter.

I breathe a sigh of relief when I see Mallory curled up with Ladybug, reading a book. She is wearing one of my favorite sweatshirts with the sleeves rolled up.

I place the scarf back in the box and close the dresser drawer. When Mallory hears me, she looks up at me with tears in her eyes. "I'm so sorry. I didn't mean to be ungrateful. I know you were trying to be nice."

Carefully, I sit on the bed next to Mallory. Ladybug wags her tail and scoots over next to me as she tries to get more attention. Mallory scoots back and tucks herself next to me against the headboard.

"What's wrong?" I probe gently.

Mallory runs her hands over the patches of hair still left on her balding head. "I can't pretend anymore."

I kiss her forehead. "You know, I'm aware that you have cancer. You never have to pretend with me."

Mallory shakes her head. "You don't understand. I know this sounds delusional but as long as I looked like I didn't have cancer, I guess I felt like I could fool myself and everyone else. This was only just a temporary setback, right? I caught it early, just a few rounds of chemo and a chunk of tissue gone and I'd be fine. But today's a wake-up call that I might not be fine. Now that I've lost my hair, every time I look in the mirror, it's a reminder that I might die."

I hug her closer. "I know it's hard. But it doesn't change anything. Doctor Stephenson and Doctor Blumenauer are still pleased with your lab results, you are healing well and responding to treatment. You've even managed to reach a truce with your nausea. Remember Doctor Stephenson said she wished all of her patients responded as well as you have?"

"I know all that. But this feels like a catastrophic setback."

"It's an unfortunate side effect of your medication, it doesn't mean you're getting worse."

Mallory puts her hands on her head and more tufts of hair fall out. "I look like a scary Halloween costume," she whispers in a tearful voice. "I don't know how you can stand to be around me these days. I look like something from a horror movie and I routinely throw up everywhere."

"Mallory, that's not who you are. That's just temporary garbage you're going through because of your treatment. All that doesn't matter to me. I see who you are on the inside and I love you. We can deal with the cosmetic stuff —"

Mallory draws in a deep breath before she blurts, "I love you too, but what if love isn't enough?"

"What do you mean?" I ask.

"There are no guarantees I'm going to get better. I watch the other patients at chemotherapy. We lost another long timer last week. It looked like he was getting better and then his body just gave up. That could happen to me! I roped you into this whole pretend husband gig. What if losing my hair is only the beginning of the end?"

"You're right there are no guarantees — but that's true for everyone. I see it every day in my job. Couples who kiss each other goodbye in the morning and one of them never comes home. The best we can do is to love with our whole heart when we are here on earth."

"What are you going to do if things don't go well with me? I feel like I've sentenced you to a life of sadness."

"That's not true, Mal. Despite the struggles with your cancer, I'm happier than I've ever been. Your cancer scares the bejeebees out of me most days — but honestly, I don't think your hair loss is a bad omen of things to come. I just think it's a side effect of the chemo."

"You are such an incurable optimist," Mallory mutters to herself.

I carefully extradite myself from the bed and run to the spare bedroom and grab my shaving kit. I stride back into Mallory's room holding up a new razor and a can of shaving cream.

"It's not in my power to eradicate your cancer cells, but I can make your side effects a little more bearable. Let's say we even out your look a little bit?"

Mallory nods with tears in her eyes. "Everybody warned me to get my hair cut short months ago so this wouldn't be so hard."

I help her off the bed and pull her close into an embrace as I kiss the top of her head. "I think it would be hard either way. Like you said, there's a whole lot of symbolism involved in this. But, we'll get through it together."

"I know I should've been ready for this. But I don't know if I'll be able to face the world looking like a pool ball with eyes," Mallory mumbles against my chest.

"I've been doing some research. It turns out someone I went to school with started a durable medical equipment company to deal with your kind of situation. I have to work for the next few days, but I would love for you to meet Iris. I think she might have the perfect solution."

Mallory lifts her head and looks me in the eye. "Solutions would be nice. I'm tired of looking at the ugly side of problems."

CHAPTER TWENTY

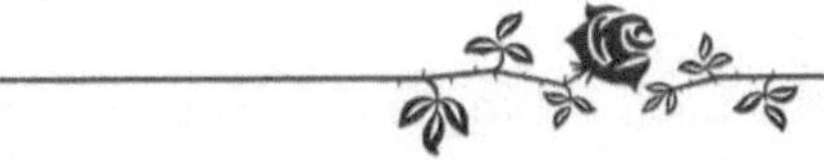

MALLORY

ROCCO HOLDS MY HAND as we walk into a shop in the historic part of town. There are mannequins with beautiful lingerie and a wall full of wigs in a variety of hairstyles and hair colors. A woman with a long caftan, sparkling blue eyes and spiky gray hair greets me with a wide smile. "Oh, what a beautiful headscarf! I just love silk. I'm Iris, how can I help you?"

"I came to ask about wigs," I mumble.

Iris clasps her hands together in front of her. "How fun! You have delightful bone structure. You could wear almost anything. Would you like to be daring or more traditional?"

I blush. "I think I'm a traditional kind of gal. Even as a teenager, I didn't experiment much with hair dye or funky hairstyles."

"So, no bright pink hair for you?" Iris teases.

Rocco shrugs. "It could be fun. You could look like a pop star."

I look around the shop. "Tempting, but not today," I

answer with a giggle. "Can you imagine what my dad would say?"

Slowly, I walk up and down the aisles of the shop. Finally, I stop in front of a wig which resembles my natural hair. It's a little shorter than I usually wear my hair, but it looks cute on the mannequin. "What about this one?"

"I have one in the back I think is just your size. A gal ordered it for her wedding and decided she wanted long hair instead."

Iris escorts us to a dressing room. Nervously, I take off the headscarf Rocco had purchased for me. I've had three days to get used to being bald. It's still shocking. Not as shocking as the first day when Rocco gently shaved off all the tufts of hair which remained after that fateful shower. I think he had almost as tough a time with it as I did. My tears nearly did him in. If I wasn't in love with him before that day, I fell in love then. When I told him so, we just held each other for hours. It wasn't how I scripted the fairytale to go when I was a little girl — but sometimes reality makes love so much more real than your dreams.

Iris comes into the dressing room with the wig. She puts an odd little covering on my scalp and then places the wig on my head. I close my eyes. I'm almost afraid to look. If I'm disappointed I don't know what my options are. After a few little tugs and flips, Iris says, "Honey, you can open your eyes. You look beautiful."

I open them cautiously, afraid of what I'll see. When I think of wigs, I think of Halloween. I never thought I'd be wearing one. My reflection comes into focus through my tears and I can't believe what I see. It looks like the me before cancer. The hair is full, shiny and bouncy. I start to cry in earnest and I have to turn around and bury my face in Rocco's chest. "I look like myself," I sob.

"I have to agree," Iris comments. "Even if I had had to custom order this wig for you, I don't think I would've changed a thing. It's perfect."

I run my fingers through the hair. "This is real human hair, isn't it? When I was researching about chemotherapy, I heard these are very expensive." I hang my head. "I may not be able to get it."

"Don't lose hope just yet. Do you have a prescription from your doctor?"

I shake my head. "It never occurred to me to get one. Does insurance even cover this kind of thing?"

Iris clicks her tongue. "In my opinion, all insurance companies should cover it — but some of them do and some of them don't. I have good luck getting them to cover it. I just need a prescription from your doctor. You should not have much trouble getting one."

"This wig is so perfect. What if you sell it before I get the paperwork in place?"

"Honey, as far as I'm concerned, the wig is yours until you tell me otherwise. It sat in my back room for quite some time; it can sit back there a little longer."

Iris carefully removes the wig and artfully ties my scarf back on my head.

Rocco sees my devastation and kisses my forehead. "Don't worry about it, that wig will be yours one way or the other. Let's go see Doctor Stephenson and get a prescription. Let me call over there and tell them we're on our way."

I walk over toward the lingerie while Rocco talks on

the phone. I encounter some bras with odd pockets in the cups. Iris follows me. "Let me know if you have any questions."

I turn toward her and shyly ask, "What are these for?"

"These are for women who need various size prosthetics. Not every woman chooses to have full mastectomies. Some women elect to have lumpectomies. Many of them find they are unhappy with the way their figure looks afterwards. So, they wear a little something in their lingerie to even things out."

"No way! I thought it was just me. I didn't want to say anything because I felt ungrateful. After all, I still have most of my breast tissue, but I feel uneven and lumpy. It's like I have a woman's breast on one side and a prepubescent adolescent's breast on the other. It's embarrassing."

"It's not just you. We all like to feel beautiful in our skin. If you don't mind me asking, where did they take your tissue from?"

I blush a little before I answer, "Mostly, from the underside of my left breast, but they took a little from my armpit as well."

Iris digs through some inventory. "You're usually about a 34B, aren't you?"

"It's pretty scary that you can guess that," I comment as I cross my arms in front of me.

"Nothing scary about it. I worked at an upscale department store for years. Measuring people for bras was what I did. Soon, I could just eyeball people — course it wasn't store policy, I still had to use a measuring tape. More often than not, I was right."

"That's an odd talent to have."

"It sure helped when they moved me to the bridal department," Iris answers with a wink. "Anyway, this model here is excellent for the type of surgery you had. See this little pocket here? It securely holds miniature silicone cutlets as we call them. There are several sizes available — so it's easy to match with your natural breast."

"Oh wow! I didn't even know they made such a thing."

"You could get a prescription for this too."

Rocco comes back into the store. "I'm on the phone with Doctor Stephenson's medical assistant. She wants to know if you also want a prescription for prosthetic lingerie."

I look to Iris for confirmation.

She turns to Rocco. "I work with Doctor Stephenson's office quite a bit. I'll get the precise insurance codes they'll need and fax it over to them."

Rocco repeats the information to the doctor's office. When he hangs up he is grinning. "They said they'll be happy to provide anything you need."

Iris looks at me and says, "Do you happen to have your insurance card on you?"

I dig through my purse and eventually find the card my dad gave me. When Iris sees it, she smiles like it's Christmas and her birthday all at once.

"Honey, it's your lucky day. Of all the insurance companies I deal with, that one is a breeze. Depending on how quickly your doctor's office and I can fax back and forth, you guys can probably go get some lunch and come back this afternoon and get your wig."

"Are you kidding me?" I exclaim, practically jumping up and down.

"Nope, I got good contacts in the claims department. Go treat yourself to a celebration lunch and we'll talk later."

<hr>

"Are you ready for this?" Rocco asks me as we walk into the ceremony.

"As ready as I'll ever be — thanks to Iris. That woman is a miracle worker. I feel like my old self — actually better than my old self. I didn't know half the stuff I needed to know about foundation garments until Iris showed me what I should wear under this dress. I love you for introducing me to her. She has made this cancer thing a lot easier for me."

"Well, whatever she taught you, you learned your lessons well. You look magnificent," he says as he leans down to brush a kiss across my lips.

"You don't look so bad yourself. I didn't realize paramedics have dress uniforms." I stand on my tiptoes to kiss him more deeply.

"We don't wear them much in public. Usually if we wear them, it's for a sad occasion like a funeral procession or something," he answers looking around the ballroom nervously.

"That's not the case tonight — you and Raylene are getting honored. I'm so proud of you!"

Rocco tugs at his collar. "Honestly, I'd much rather be honored for another call, almost any other call. It feels strange to get a commendation for this one. We lost a kid on this one — a twin even. It doesn't seem fair."

"You don't have to talk to me about life not being fair. But you and Raylene went above and beyond the call of duty. The minivan was on fire when you rescued the little boy and his mom. That deserves recognition. The boy who was killed was gone before you even got there. Deep down inside, you know it was too late for him. The drunk driver decimated his side of the van."

"In my head, I know that. Even so, it just seems wrong to celebrate a partial victory."

He tries not to let his nerves show as Raylene and I chat back and forth over dinner. We're having fun exchanging stories about what annoys us about Rocco. We're just having fun, but Rocco looks a bit pained about the direction of our conversation. Then Raylene shows me pictures of her kids on her cell phone and I reciprocate with goofy pictures of Chevy Chase and Ladybug as if they are our real kids. In an instant, a random thought crosses my mind. I wonder if we'll be doing the same thing in a few years with our own children.

Before I can get too emotional over my random thoughts, the Fire Chief calls Raylene and Rocco up to the stage. I cheer like they're a pair of rock stars. Rocco looks shocked when the mother of the twins comes up to give a heartfelt speech about how grateful she was for their intervention and how happy she is that they were able to save at least one of her boys. By the time she's done with her speech half the audience is wiping their eyes with napkins. Before she hands Rocco the plaque, she hugs him and whispers in his ear, "You have to forgive yourself for what you weren't able to do and be thankful for what you did do. You saved our lives. Because of you, my husband still has a family."

Fortunately for all of us, her words were picked up by the microphone and broadcast.

"Thank you. I'm glad to see you doing so well," he says as he returns her hug.

When Rocco walks back to the table, I stand up and kiss him. "See? Even when you don't think you're perfect, you're perfect in someone's eyes. I love you Rocco Pierce. You're my hero. I hope someday you'll stop being my pretend husband and be my real one."

When I arrive for my chemotherapy treatment there is a pall over the whole department. Everywhere I look someone is crying. My heart drops to my toes. Frantically I search for Sheila. As far as I know, she is the most ill among all of our regulars. My search is brought to an abrupt halt when I see her hugging some of the monopoly players.

Sheila turns and looks at me with a teary smile. "Wow! You look like a million dollars. I can see you've had the 'I've-got-cancer-but-cancer-doesn't-have-me' makeover."

Following Sheila's lead to stick with a lighthearted conversation, I curtsy. "Yeah, Rocco found all the stuff for me. Somebody finally taught me how to use makeup appropriately. You would think I'd know how to do it by now. I'm almost thirty. At any rate, I'm starting to feel like my old self."

"Good for you! You might've heard, I've decided today is the end of the road for me. I talked to my sister, and she's okay with it. Stella doesn't want me to hurt anymore. She came with me to my last appointment with my oncologist — she understands now. My dad is upset, but you know, this isn't about him. It's all about ego. But his ego can't beat my cancer. I'm done torturing my body."

Tears spring to my eyes. I know better than most what she's going through, but it still sucks. Sheila is too young to die. Cancer doesn't give a rat's butt about that.

I take a couple of moments to find my words. "What happens next?" I finally whisper in a broken voice.

"I go home and hope my appetite comes back, so I can eat all the stuff I like because I don't have to worry about getting fat anymore. I hang out with my little sis and try to teach her a lifetime of lessons in however long I have left. If my dad isn't a complete jerk about things, I might try to patch up our relationship, so he doesn't regret what could have been. When the pain becomes unbearable, I'll check myself into hospice, so I don't make my family suffer any more than they need to."

"Is there anything I can do?"

"I don't know. Can you fix my past?"

"I'm working on it. Do you want to talk to me in the headache room while I get my treatment? There have been a few developments."

"I have to say a few more goodbyes while you get situated, but I'll join you when I can."

***

Gemma's mascara is running a little as she hooks up my medication. "Are you okay?" I ask gently.

"No, not really — I may not be for a while. You

would think I'd get used to the loss by now. I've been a nurse long enough, I should develop some sort of calluses against this kind of thing — but I never do. I take each defeat personally."

"I think I would be the same way. I haven't known Sheila very long, but it already feels like a profound loss."

Gemma nods. "But like Sheila said, sometimes the bravest decision is knowing when to call it quits. At least she's doing it on her terms."

"I hope if I'm ever in her shoes, I can be equally brave."

"Now, don't you go thinking that way. Your situation is completely different from Sheila's. You can beat your cancer," Gemma reprimands sternly.

"I know the odds are in my favor. But, there's still a statistical chance I might not."

"Doctor Blumenauer is no fool. He'll track your progress with blood work and imaging. He won't let it get as advanced as Sheila's. You caught it early and it's being managed by one of the best teams around. You'll be one of our success stories. I can tell you're a fighter. Don't let the failure of another patient's treatment regimen derail you."

Sheila sticks her head around the corner. "Yeah, listen to her. You've got too much important stuff to do with your life. I knew going into treatment, it wouldn't work. Everybody knew. I just wasn't strong enough to say no. It took meeting my friends and the staff here to give me the sense of autonomy I needed to stand up for what I knew was right. Part of that meant telling the whole story about Marshall Todd but the other part of it meant leveling with Stella and not shielding her from the truth of how sick I really was. Now, I'm truly free."

Tears are flowing down Gemma's face. As I gather up my tubing and stand up to leave, I give her a one-armed hug. "Sheila and I have some unfinished business to discuss in the headache room. If you need it for another patient, just let me know."

As I push my IV pole down the hall, Sheila remarks, "It's beyond strange just to walk down the hall. This will sound stupid — but this place has become my home. I'm much more comfortable here than I am at my real home. I don't know what I'll do without my friends. I don't think they're allowed to just let me hang out if I'm not getting treatment."

"Well, you won't get rid of me quite so easily. I'm going to give you my contact information. You better get in touch. Besides, I have to tell you my boyfriend has the coolest friends ever. I've never seen anything like it. Some of them are famous people."

Sheila's eyes widen "Like legit famous people? Like I'd know who they are?"

"Totally. I was shocked. They act like totally normal people. I even asked them about being tabloid fodder. They said it was life. In fact, one of them is related to one of the reporters. It's too weird."

"And you think these people would want to hang out with somebody like me? I have cancer and I only have one leg, remember?"

"Something tells me, it won't matter to this particular group of people. Among that gang, neither of those things makes you unique," I quip as I sit down in the oversized reclining chair and pull my computer out of my bag.

"What do you mean?"

"Well, besides me there are three other people who have battled cancer. Madison's husband is an amputee and Mindy's mom is in a wheelchair. I think she was in some sort of accident as a child. Mindy's fiancé has Tourette's syndrome and her uncle is deaf."

"That's a pretty rad crew. I may have to take you up on your offer."

When Sheila sees my computer, she sobers. "You said there were some developments in Marshall Todd's case."

"I had a chance to meet with Marshall Todd to discuss his case."

Sheila pales. "You did? How is he? Is he okay?"

"It's funny, he asked me almost the same exact questions about you."

Sheila looks perplexed. "He did? I figured he would still be cursing my name — after all, I'm the reason he is in jail."

"Make no mistake, he's not happy about that. He doesn't understand your testimony. But I got the impression he liked you."

"Like, liked me — as in had a crush on me?" she asks incredulously.

I smile. "I'm no expert, but it seemed like that to me. That's why your testimony was even more devastating to him. He thought the two of you were friends."

"Does he understand I wish I could go back and rewrite history? If I knew back then about the strength I have now, I would've never caved to my parent's ideas about what I should have done. I would have insisted on a rape kit and a lie detector test and anything else I could've done."

"I got the sense he understood what it meant to sacrifice for your sister. He has a little brother. He said he would do almost anything for him too."

"I know this is selfish of me, but did he say anything about forgiving me for what I did?"

"It might be a little early for that. I think he was just trying to absorb everything we were telling him. We were giving him a lot of information. I think with time to process everything he'll probably come around. It's difficult for him to hope things in his life will change at this point. After all, he was convicted of a crime he didn't commit. It should not have even been a close call."

Sheila hangs her head. "I wish there was some way I could serve out my hospice time in jail and let him go free. That's what should happen."

"I don't think it works that way." I reach out and squeeze her hand. "You've done what you can do. We'll take it from here."

"What'll happen now?"

"I'll write up what I know. Andre, my assistant, is working on finding other witnesses who are willing to sign affidavits. My friend Tyler, who is a Sheriff in a different county, is sifting through law enforcement accounts and getting videotapes from the case. When we have it all together, we'll go to the law enforcement authorities and try again with the new information. Together, we'll go to the DA. I understand there's a new District Attorney now. If all goes well, she might agree to ask the court to overturn the verdict."

"What if I don't live long enough to testify?" Sheila

asks as she rubs her temples.

"I'm sure they'll make allowances for your health. The attorneys might take a videotaped deposition or something. That's why I'm working on this as quickly as I possibly can."

Sheila's expression grows resolute as she says sternly, "Promise me one thing. Don't compromise your health to fix my past. It's not worth it."

"I promise. I have a blindingly bright future to live for. I'll be diligent but cautious."

I take a business card out of my computer case and hand it to Sheila. "I meant what I said. For as long as you are able, please keep in touch."

Chapter Twenty-One

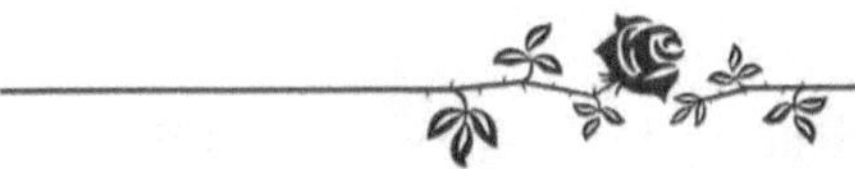

Rocco

My protective mask makes my face itch as I flip through the channels on the TV looking for something to watch. "I've forgotten how spoiled I am by DVR," I grumble when I can't find the game I'm looking for.

Mallory pushes her iPad toward me. "Maybe you can find it on here. I think you can play back everything we've recorded at home."

"Just forget it," I say as I pace around the room.

"You might as well just go to the wedding. Mindy and Elijah want you there. It's not their fault my blood count went crazy," Mallory insists. "My oncologist said it would be at least three more days before he could spring me. He doesn't want to switch me to oral antibiotics. Besides, they are trying me on a new medication for my nerve pain. They want to observe my reaction to it."

I scrub my hand down my face. "I don't want to leave you behind. You were looking forward to the wedding."

Mallory points to her beeping IV monitor, the oximeter clamped to her finger, and the oxygen cannula in her nose. "Well, I didn't plan on cancer wiping out my immune system either. But crap happens. Elijah wants you to be part of his big day. So, you should be there."

"I had plans for that wedding," I pout.

A ghost of a smile passes over Mallory's lips. "Believe it or not, so did I. But, like everything else lately, it doesn't seem to matter what I plan."

"Go and tell Heather her cake is beautiful and take lots of pictures of Mindy and Elijah. I know they'll be a stunning couple. I'll be fine here. The nurses here are great. Sheila even said she might stop by for old time's sake if she's feeling well enough."

I start to remove my protective clothing.

"What are you doing?" Mallory asks with a somewhat panicked expression.

"I'll be right back. I forgot something in my glove box."

"Can't it wait?"

"Not if I'm leaving. I promise, I'll be right back."

"Please tell me it's not a puppy. I mean, I love our little menagerie. But we can't handle another animal."

I laugh out loud. "No, I swear it is not another animal. Although, Raylene and I responded to a house fire the other day and they were rescuing a hedgehog. The family said they couldn't take it to the shelter, and they were looking for someone to take it. I was mighty tempted."

Mallory pulls the blanket up around her neck. "I know you mean well Rocco, but I think we have our hands full."

"I understand, but you have no idea how cute the

hedgehog was. If you would've been there, you would've been tempted too."

"Probably — that's why it's a good thing I wasn't there with you."

I touch Mallory's cheek as I walk by. I miss being able to kiss her, but for now, it's a risk I just can't take.

When I come back in the room and put on new protective clothing, Mallory's expression is anxious. "What's wrong?"

"I thought maybe I upset you," she admits.

"No, that's not it at all. It has more to do with the abrupt change of plans. If things had played out the way we had hoped, we would be over on the beautiful Oregon coast at William Gardner's beach house celebrating with our friends."

Mallory's shoulders hunch and she appears dejected. "I'm sorry I ruined all that. You really should go. Your friends are like family to you."

I reach into my jacket pocket. "No, you misunderstand. That's not what this conversation is about at all. I just wanted to do this in a more picturesque setting with our friends and family around. But, since I can't, this will have to do —"

Mallory's eyes widen and she scrambles to get out of bed. "Oh no you don't!" she says as she tries to run toward the cupboard where she stores her purse. "This is not how I planned for this to happen either. I had plans for this weekend too. It's your birthday." She tries to balance against her IV pole and reach through the wires as she digs through her purse. Triumphantly, she comes up with a box.

"Me first," she demands as she awkwardly balances

against the IV pole and kneels in front of me. She opens a ring box. "Rocco Alexander Pierce, when you first suggested being my pretend husband to help me through the most difficult time in my life, I thought you were a little crazy, to be honest. But then I discovered what an amazing man you really are. Second by second, day by day I fell a little more in love with you. Rocco Pierce will you marry me for real? I will love you for better and for worse and obviously in sickness and in health and in times of sadness and in great joy for as long as we both shall live."

As many ways as I rehearsed this day in my head, this was not one of them. I help Mallory to her feet as she slides the ring on to my finger. I pull my mask down a little and kiss her on the cheek. "Nariko Yoshida or Mallory Edmondson or whatever you choose to call yourself, I would be honored to be your husband. I love you. I think I have since the day we met."

Kneeling down on one knee, I open the ring box and take the ring out. "It seems we often have the same great ideas. Mallory, I have had the best time of my life pretending to be your husband. I would love to make our arrangement permanent. Would you do me the honor of becoming the real Mrs. Pierce?"

"Any day you choose. Mr. Pierce, I love you," Mallory exclaims as she reaches down and tries to help me to my feet. I slide the simple silver band on her finger.

We compare our bands and find them remarkably similar. I raise an eyebrow. "Gee, I wonder how that happened?"

We look at each other and simultaneously guess, "Mindy?"

"I didn't talk to her about rings, did you?" Mallory

insists.

I shake my head. "Me neither. I actually didn't talk to anybody."

"That's just spooky," Mallory says as a shiver goes up her spine.

"I guess we just chalk this up to another example of how utterly compatible we are."

"I suppose so. I'm a little scared to contemplate anything else."

"I guess if I'm going to go to the wedding, I should probably get going. Maybe I can catch a ride with Toby."

"That's a great idea. I'll still be your fiancée when you get back." Mallory teases. She pretends to blow me a kiss.

I pretend to catch it. Yet, I regret not being able to pull off some grand gesture people will talk about for years to come.

Mallory catches my crushed expression.

She runs her hand down my face. "Trust me, this was perfect. I'll remember it forever."

———•———

Mallory whips her head set off when she sees me standing in the doorway and she almost drops her computer. "What are you doing here? Mindy and Elijah are supposed to get married *today*. The wedding is on the coast!"

I start to put the protective clothing and mask on and Mallory waves me off. "Guess what? My blood panels are within normal range so the doctor said none of that was necessary unless the person coming to see me is ill. You're not sick, are you?"

I shake my head. "No, I feel fine. Actually, I'm better than fine today. The new rules will make things exponentially easier."

"That doesn't explain why you're here instead of there," Mallory presses. "What things?"

Mindy pokes her head around the corner. She is still wearing her veil and her wedding dress.

"Mindy!" Mallory shrieks. "What are you doing here?" She looks up at the clock. "You are supposed to be walking down the aisle right about now."

Mindy waves the rest of the people into Mallory's room. Fortunately, we are frequent enough flyers around here they've learned to give Mallory a large room. Between her family, my family, her coworkers and random neighbors, it's almost always a full house.

Mallory watches with wide-eyed astonishment as Justice Gardner, his wife Isobel, Aidan O'Brien and Tara, Jeff and Keira, Tyler and Heather, Elijah's parents and Tasha and Jude pour into the room. "What's going on?" Mallory stammers.

"The paparazzi didn't listen to Howard's misdirection this time. So, they swarmed William and Isobel's place. We couldn't get a moment's peace. So, we decided to bring the wedding to you."

"You want to have your wedding in my hospital room?" Mallory sounds as flabbergasted as I did when they first ran the idea past me.

Elijah nods. "Jigger, jig, jig, you were part of the reason I was brave enough to ask Mindy to marry me that night. Jigger, jig, jig, you shouldn't have to miss our wedding just because your body is busy fighting cancer."

I open and close my mouth as if I'm a guppy. "Umm,

okay. But we haven't been friends all that long." I stammer as I try to absorb it all.

"Sometimes, it's not about how long you have been friends with someone, but rather the quality of experiences you've shared," Elijah adds philosophically.

Heather grins. "Besides, it's kind of a Girlfriend Posse tradition to ditch the paparazzi at weddings. I have to say though, this particular ditching is a thing of beauty. It'll be awhile before this one is topped."

Mindy giggles. "I know. Uncle Aidan and Aunt Tara thought they pulled off the greatest paparazzi fake out ever — but Elijah and I may be the new record holders."

Kiera smiles up at Mallory. "So, what do you say? Can we borrow your room to get my daughter married to the love of her life?"

Mallory's brows furrow. "Are you sure you want to? There are some beautiful parks around — they would have much better scenery for pictures."

Elijah steps up toward the head of Mallory's bed. "Jigger, jig, jig, that could be true — and pictures are nice. But that's not what we're about. Mindy and I both live our lives in the spotlight. People take pictures whether we want them to or not. What we care about is sharing our love story with the people who mean the most to us."

"How can I be one of those people? We just met a few months ago."

"You believed in me and the power of love when I was a little too nervous to have the faith I needed, jigger, jig, jig. That means the world to us. Mindy and I could have gotten married anywhere — quite literally. But we chose to have our service here so you could be part of it."

Mallory picks up a Kleenex from her bedside table and starts dabbing at the corners of her eyes.

"Darn it! You guys have me crying like a baby over here. When I first moved to Oregon, I was afraid. I was sure I wouldn't have any friends or family to call my own. With your help, I have laid claim to both."

Justice Gardner clears his throat. "Maybe this might be a good time to get started."

Mallory's hands fly up to her head which is now covered in a thin layer of peach fuzz. "Mindy, I can't be in your wedding pictures like this. I look awful."

Mindy looks around at her family and friends. "You know what? It's been a crazy day. I know you guys must be starving. Why don't you guys go to Papa and Grummy's house for a bite to eat while we get everything situated here? Aunt Donda is on her way. She and Jaxson just had to ditch some paparazzi first."

Mallory looks at Mindy in confusion. "Donda beats me at pool all the time, but what does she have to do with how awful I look?"

Mindy giggles. "I forgot, you haven't been to a kajillion of our weddings around here. But Aunt Donda and my dad are like the go-to glam team. Do you have your wig here? My dad can put all sorts of fancy braids in it for you."

"I was wearing it when I was admitted. I collapsed at work because I didn't realize how sick I was. I think I'll skip the braids, thanks anyway. I could definitely use some makeup though. Unfortunately, I don't have any with me."

Kiera smirks. "I think you underestimate the power of my sister-in-law. She does everyone's makeup at our shindigs. She'll have you covered. Don't worry about it. She'll be excited to have a new victim to work on."

"Should I be scared?" Mallory asks.

Isobel steps forward. "No, you most definitely should not be scared. It was an unfortunate choice of words. Donda is very talented. I look forward to all the weddings this group has because Donda always makes me feel quite glamorous."

Mallory shoots me a panicked gaze. I walk over to her side and hold her hand. Squatting down next to the head of her bed, I whisper, "Are you all right with all of this? I know we kind of dumped it on you suddenly. You don't have to do it if you don't feel up to it."

Mallory gestures around at all the medical equipment and her hospital gown. "I want to be part of Mindy's special day. She's come to mean a lot to me. But I don't want her to regret the decision to include me."

Elijah's mom shakes her head. "Don't you worry. They're not the kind of people to care about that kind of thing, are they Seth?" she confirms with Elijah's dad. He shakes his head.

Mindy comes over to the side of the bed. "You know, there was a time in my life when I used to think weddings had to go exactly as planned in order to be perfect. But along the way, I grew up and realized it wasn't what happened at a wedding that counted; it was who was involved in your life and what they meant to you. It's not about the pictures, dresses, or the cake." She looks hastily over her shoulder at Heather. "Sorry, Aunt Heather."

Heather just laughs. "It's okay, Mindy Mouse. I make wedding cakes for a living and I still agree with you."

"What I mean is it doesn't matter if my wedding isn't

at the beach, or in a beautiful church. It matters that the friends I care about are here."

"Does that clear things up?" I ask as I wipe a tear from Mallory's cheek.

She nods. "Now, get out of here. We've got to get beautified for this thing. By the way, bring me back one of Gwendolyn's lemon scones. I'm starving. I've been living on hospital food way too long."

I bow as I back away from the bed. "Would you like anything else, my dear fiancée? A latte or chai tea, perhaps?"

"My grandma makes the best chai tea. Vote for that!" Mindy instructs enthusiastically.

Mallory chuckles. "Okay, I guess you have your marching orders."

⚊⚫⚊

When I reenter Mallory's hospital room, it bears little resemblance to the place I left earlier. Flower blossoms and white Christmas lights are strung around the room. Light acoustic music is playing in the background. My fiancée looks nothing like the frail woman who was lying in the bed before. She is sitting up with Aidan and Tara's daughter, Maddie, on her lap playing a game on the iPad.

She blushes when she sees my open perusal. "They were right, Donda is a miracle worker."

To me, Mallory is always beautiful, but Donda has highlighted her beautiful eyes and cupid bow lips. Even her wig has been styled to resemble the updos Tasha and Madison are wearing. She looks sophisticated and a little sultry at the same time. My heart skips a beat. I can't believe I'm so lucky. Someday soon, I'll be in Elijah's shoes.

Mallory shifts Maddie on her lap and grimaces when the little girl inadvertently catches her IV tubing with her foot. It's a grim reminder that as much as we dress everything up, everything isn't perfect yet.

"It helps that she had a beautiful canvas to work with." I respond as I lean down and kiss her on her cheek.

Jaxson elbows me in the side. "All these years I've known you and I had no idea you were such a Romeo."

I stand up and wink. "All I needed was the proper inspiration."

Justice Gardner clears his throat. "I have done all sorts of ceremonies with this particular group of people. I have to say, this ranks as one of the most unusual. Mindy, you are the one person I expected to have a traditional, by-the-book wedding," he finishes with a laugh.

Mindy blushes as she takes Elijah's hand. "Let's say my definition of perfect has relaxed a little over the years."

Justice Gardner's eyebrows furrow. "Am I to take that to mean all the beautiful vows we rehearsed the other day are out the window?"

Mindy stands on her tiptoes and kisses the judge's cheek. "I'm afraid so, William. We're stripping it down to the basics."

"How basic?" he asks skeptically.

"Jigger, jig, jig, I just want everyone to know how much I love Mindy and I want her to be my wife," Elijah says.

"And I want everyone to know it doesn't matter what

happens in my career, Elijah is the center of my universe until the stars fall from the sky," Mindy adds. "I will love him forever."

Justice Gardner nods. "Did you guys bring rings?"

Charlie steps forward. "Yeah, they have rings. Guess what? They let me hold them. They said I was responsible enough."

The older man looks down at Charlie. "Now would be a good time for you to give the rings to Elijah and your sister."

"Now?" Charlie asks, his voice rising to a squeak at the end.

The judge smiles. "I guess this is called rolling with the punches. Nothing is going according to plan. Therefore, we're just making it up as we go along."

Charlie grins. "Oh, you mean like when Elijah-n-me make up stories for our books?"

"Sort of like that, yes," Justice Gardner answers with a deep chuckle.

Charlie dutifully hands the rings to his sister and Elijah.

The judge looks at the groom. "I think you know what to do."

Elijah slides the ring on Mindy's hand. "Jigger, jig, jig, I give you this ring as a symbol of my love and faithfulness. Our love has no beginning and no end, jigger, jig, jig. I will love you until there are no more tomorrows."

Mindy takes Elijah's ring and slides it on his finger. With her other hand, she wipes away tears. "Before I met you, I saw no one in my future. I was certain I would die alone. You are my forever happily ever after. Elijah Fischer, I give you this ring as a symbol of my love and faithfulness. Our love has been destined from the beginning of time and I will love you until time ceases to exist. As our rings say, I will love you until." Mindy's hands shake as she holds Elijah's hands in her own.

"By the power vested in me as a former officer of the court in the state of Oregon, I pronounce Mindy Jo Whitaker and Elijah Fischer to be husband and wife." Justice Gardner takes a moment to get a handkerchief out of his pocket and wipe tears from his eyes. "From the moment you came into our lives Mindy, I knew fate had something phenomenal in store for you. I'm glad you found it in this extraordinary young man who is now your husband. This may be the most unusual ceremony I've ever officiated, but it might very well be one of my favorites. You may kiss your husband, Mindy Mouse."

The room erupts in the sign language equivalent of applause so we don't disrupt the other patients.

Mallory leans her head against my arm as she whispers, "I'm so glad you didn't give up and continued to look for me. You have the coolest friends on the whole planet."

Mindy breaks away from Elijah's surprisingly theatrical kiss and looks over her shoulder at Mallory.

"I think you're pretty cool too. Just wait and see what we have in store for *your* wedding."

Chapter Twenty-Two

Mallory

I TRY TO HIDE my horrified reaction when I walk into Sheila's room. Unfortunately, I'm not a very good actress and she catches on quickly.

"It's all right. I know I'm dying. It's not a newsflash. After all, I'm in hospice. That's what you're supposed to do here." She smiles weakly.

I set down the gift bag and reach over to give her a hug. Sheila is nothing but skin and bones. She has dark circles under her eyes and she's ghostly pale. "Hey, whatever happened to the plan of eating nothing but junk food? I thought you were planning to binge on homemade macaroni and cheese and lasagna."

Sheila coughs and struggles to catch her breath. "Yeah, that was the plan — but it turns out pain medication makes me almost as sick as chemo did. Of course, it doesn't help when the cancer decides to spread everywhere."

My stomach rolls from sensory memory. I will never forget the hours I spent throwing up. "Is there anything

I can do?" I ask, but I can't help but feel my question is incredibly lame, given the circumstances.

"There isn't a lot anyone can do. Basically, they have me on as much anti-nausea medicine as I can tolerate. They've offered me a feeding tube but that kind of defeats the purpose since I'm here to die. When I get too tired of coping with it, I ask for more pain medication so I sleep through the nausea."

Sheila tries to smile brightly as she picks up the gift bag. "Did you bring me presents?"

I nod as I blink back tears. "I did. I figured you were probably bored with TV. A friend of a friend, Haley, who had Ewing's sarcoma, swears coloring makes everything better."

"That's awesome. I'll have to try it — because if I have to watch any more reality TV, I think I will go insane."

Sheila takes a look at the coloring book and the pens. "Look at these pictures! They even have your favorite cherry blossoms. How did you know to get me metallic pens?"

I shrug. "I guess I figured it was a natural match. You've always shone a little brighter than the rest of us."

"I think that's the nicest thing anyone's ever said about me," Sheila says, choking back tears.

I dig through my purse and pull out an envelope. "I'm glad you like it, but it's not the coolest thing I brought you today."

I can't hold back my emotion as I hand her the envelope.

With shaking hands, Sheila pulls out the single sheet

of paper and reads it. She starts to cry and reads it again.

"Does this say what I think it says?" she asks as she looks up at me.

"Yes, this is the statement from the new District Attorney asking for Marshall Todd's conviction to be overturned and that he not be retried. Both sides have met with the judge in the case and he is expected to honor the request."

"Are you saying this will be over?"

"It looks like it. Of course, we won't know for sure until all the paperwork is signed and Marshall Todd walks out of jail — but all indications are this fight is over. You did it!"

Sheila slumps back against her pillow. Tears are flowing out of the corners of her eyes and down onto the pillow. She struggles to set the bed up and take a drink of water. She looks at me directly and asks, "How is your battle going?"

"I had a scare a while back from something as stupid as a cold. But things are looking fantastic now. My blood work is normal, all the pathology looks great. My mammography and ultrasound were as good as they could be under the circumstances. Of course, they can't declare me to be cancer free for several more years — I seem to have beaten breast cancer into submission."

"And things with your pretend husband?" She asks as she starts to fall to the side.

Scooting closer to the bed I prop up her pillows before I hold up my engagement ring. "I decided I liked his job performance so well, I wanted him to apply for the job permanently," I tease.

"Was his proposal totally romantic?"

"You could say that, I guess. We asked each other at the same time. He was going to give me a ring, but I beat him to the punch."

Sheila laughs. "How thoroughly modern of you! How did your knight in shining armor deal with that little development?"

"He waited his turn like the gentleman he is," I answer with a grin.

Sheila coughs so hard, she begins to throw up in the little blue bag she was holding in her lap. The sound of her retching brings back so many painful memories for me I have to look away. When she's done, she calls for the nurse. The exertion leaves her breathless.

The nurse silently gives her a wet washcloth and her toothbrush. When Sheila is finished, she looks at me with the most anguished expression I've ever seen. "Mallory, I'm so tired."

"I understand. I remember how exhausting all of that is," I comment as I gently squeeze her hand.

She closes her eyes and takes a shallow breath. "No, I'm just tired of it all."

"I don't think anybody blames you, Sheila. Everyone understands you've fought an incredible battle."

"No more battles to fight, thanks to you," Sheila says as she exhales.

"I didn't do much. You are the hero," I whisper as I rub my thumb across the back of her hand.

"Only because you let me." Sheila's speech fades away. Her eyes close and everything is still.

I watch for a moment, hoping against hope what I know is true is somehow a figment of my imagination.

But, even as I pray, I know it's too late. My friend is gone. Cancer won this round.

Carefully, I remove the letter from the District Attorney from beside Sheila and tuck it back in my purse. It is a tangible reminder of why Sheila fought as long as she did.

———————◆———————

As they always are, Sheila Taylor's celebration of life is a profoundly sad affair mixed with bursts of happiness and moments of levity. I'm profoundly moved by the number of people from the center where we received our chemotherapy treatments. There are dozens and dozens of patients, nurses, administrators and even doctors here to pay their respects to Sheila. Some of them brought copies of her favorite magazines and movie posters. Others brought decks of cards and her favorite slippers.

Rocco is quietly rubbing my lower back as I sit in the pew of the church nervously waiting my turn. I turn and whisper in his ear, "I don't know if I can do this."

"You can," he replies. "Stella asked you to, and it's what Sheila would've wanted."

"I don't do this kind of thing," I hiss under my breath.

"I know you don't, but today you can. It's for Sheila."

The minister nods at me. I stand up and smooth my black dress down. I run my hand through my short pixie hairstyle. I swallow hard as I struggle to find my voice in front of all these people. But then I realize most of these people are my friends. Friends I never imagined I would make — but friends, nonetheless.

I clear my throat before I adjust the microphone

down to my height. "I thought I knew who Sheila Taylor was long before I met her. I had read hundreds of pages of news stories, school records and court transcripts. I thought I knew who she was. Honestly, I had pegged her as a coward. Someone who had wrongly accused someone of a crime. I wasn't sure why — I thought maybe she was looking to get famous or maybe she wanted to extort money from his family. Either way, I was pretty certain I didn't like Sheila Taylor."

Sheila's father stands up in the back of the room and shouts, "How dare you say any of that stuff about my daughter. Don't you respect the dead?"

Stella stands up and pulls her father back down into his seat. "Oh shut up, Dad! It's not like you haven't said that and tons of other things that were a million times worse about Sheila. You know there's more to the story. Let her tell it!"

I smile gratefully at Stella. "You're right, there is more to the story — much more. As Sheila and I both learned the hard way, life has a way of surprising you when you least expect it. I was diagnosed with breast cancer. Unlike Sheila, I was lucky. I was diagnosed incredibly early because I did a favor for a friend."

"Lucky you," grouses Sheila's dad.

"Shh!" Stella whispers.

"No, if I were in your shoes, I would feel the same way. In fact, as Sheila's friend, some days I wonder why I am cancer free and she lost her battle. Anyway, my very first day of chemotherapy, Sheila reached out to me to help teach me the ropes. Of course, then I didn't know who she was. But after she introduced herself, I had to reconcile who I thought she was with the person sitting in the chair across from me fighting the same battle."

I swallow hard and take a drink of water from the bottle sitting on the podium.

"At first, I wondered if I should even tell her who I was or that I knew anything about her past. Yet, I decided ethically I had a duty to say something. So I did. I was afraid she wouldn't talk to me anymore. I was surprised when she not only talked to me, but she was brutally honest about her role in the imprisonment of Marshall Todd. She made it her mission to set the record straight and try to get his conviction overturned before she passed away."

I draw in a deep breath and wipe my eyes before I continue. "Unfortunately, we're not quite there yet. But I was able to unearth enough evidence to convince the DA to recommend that the conviction be set aside and Marshall Todd not be retried. At this point, it looks like the judge's signature is a mere formality. So, the young woman I thought was a coward who didn't care about justice fought until the very end to do the right thing, fix a miscarriage of justice, and set a man free. I am honored to have called Sheila Taylor my friend and I will miss her as I know all of you will."

As I turn to leave the stage, Stella runs up on stage and gives me a hug. "Thank you, thank you so much. You don't know the gift you gave my sister. You may not have been able to cure her cancer or make her pain go away, but you gave her a voice — a voice she hadn't had in almost a decade. Even though she was ravaged by cancer, exercising her voice gave her a sense of freedom no words can explain. Thank you for believing in my sister."

I hold Stella close as I whisper, "That belief went both ways. Sheila believed that together we could change the world, so we did. She believes in you too."

"I know. I'm going to go to law school to help people like Marshall Todd. I think Sheila would really like that."

"I know she would. She was so proud of you."

Epilogue

Rocco

My mom always used to say she was bursting her buttons with pride whenever Remy or I did something noteworthy in school or on the athletic field. Until tonight, I never understood the meaning of the phrase. Yet, looking at Mallory all dressed up on stage with other journalists from all around the world, I get it now.

Marshall leans over and asks, "You think she's nervous?"

Before I get a chance to say a word, Andre chuckles. "I hope she's wearing an adult diaper. If I know my boss, she's getting ready to pee her pants. She hates this kind of stuff."

"Maybe so, but without her writing, I don't think I would be sitting here beside you. I owe that woman my life," Marshall insists.

"Yeah, she's a heckuva writer. But, if you ask her, she'll tell you she's not winning this award because of her journalism skills, she'll say it's all the work of Sheila and she was just the vessel to make sure justice is done in a case where it was overlooked before," Andre replies.

"All I can say is I met with a lot of reporters over the years and nobody cared enough to find out the real truth. Mallory is the only one who dug to the bottom of the case, even before she met Sheila, to find out what was really going on. I guess you can say I'm grateful to both of them. I wish I could have told Sheila in person before she passed away."

The pain in Marshall's face hits me hard in the gut. I could easily be in his shoes if Mallory's cancer hadn't been found early or if I hadn't been able to locate her, or even if the screw-up hadn't happened and no one had notified her of her cancer.

"Mallory spent a lot of time talking to Sheila. I'm sure she told her how grateful you were she came forward and did the right thing. That's just the kind of person Mallory is."

"She told me how the two of you met. Did you guys ever think about suing the hospital? Seems to me somebody should be held responsible for something like that," Marshall suggests.

Andre reaches out and gives Marshall a high five. "I told her the same thing! She told me to mind my own business!"

I chuckle. "At first, I was upset. After all, how could they be so negligent? After a while, I decided maybe it wasn't negligence after all. Maybe it was simply a flat-out miracle that brought Mallory and I together. There is no logical explanation for what happened, so I have to chalk it up to the hand of fate, God, or a miracle — and just be thankful I was the one to get those records and find the love of my life."

Jaxson taps me on the shoulder. "I hate to break up this mush fest, but you all might want to pay attention to what's happening on stage —"

"... and this year's Impact Award for Outstanding Achievement in Online Journalism goes to Mallory Yoshida. She is being recognized for her in-depth reporting on a case that had disappeared from social media and the front pages of the news. The people in the story could've easily been forgotten were it not for the efforts of Ms. Yoshida. Because of her excellent reporting, a wrongful conviction was overturned, and the defendant was released and reunited with his family. The real story was told and to the extent possible, a wrong was made right. The editorial board for this award had a chance to meet with Ms. Yoshida. I have to tell you, she is one of the most reluctant winners we have ever had. Not because she is ashamed of the work she did. She is not. She is proud to have helped restore some justice in a case where there was very little. But she wants the credit to go where it belongs — to a witness who at the time of the trial had very few choices and felt that her voice was being ignored. That witness chose to come forward and push for the truth to be told. Ms. Yoshida insists her role was quite minimal. We'll let you decide. I present to you Mallory Yoshida, winner of the Impact Award for Outstanding Achievement in Online Journalism."

Mallory steps forward and tucks her hair behind her ear. "First, I'd like to thank my fellow journalists for this award. It means the world to me. You'll all be very thankful that this speech is quite short. The last time I had to give a speech I rambled on for what seemed like forever. I just want to thank my colleagues at *Word Soup, PNW* for sticking beside me when things got dicey there for a while. Cancer is no joke. I want to thank Andre for being the best assistant ever."

Andre gives a large fist pump. "Woot, I got a shout out!" he exclaims under his breath.

"Even though she's no longer here, I want to thank Sheila Taylor for sticking to her guns and telling the truth even when it was hard. I want to thank Marshall Todd for being gracious under circumstances under which most of us would be anything but."

Marshall scrunches down in his seat hoping no one will notice.

"Last, I'd like to thank my fiancé and all of his phenomenal friends for being there for me in countless ways. Without your support, I'm not sure this story would've ever come together. Rocco Pierce, I thank God every day for the letter — even though it contained the scariest news of my life."

I grin like a fool and give her a huge thumbs up sign as I mouth the words, 'I love you too! I can't wait to be your husband for real.'

Note from the Author

Dear Reader,

Thanks for giving my book a read. If you liked reading about people who struggle with unique problems, you'll love what's coming.

Will Kordes has fought his whole life to be respected. He never fit in anywhere, even as a kid. It seems his brain just wired differently. Labeled a troublemaker early, he has fought the stigma for as long as he can remember.

He's not dumb, obstinate or delinquent — he just sees the world from a different angle. He thought things would be different when he sold one of his inventions for an obscene amount of money.

Will sets out to change the world, unfortunately when he meets someone who really matters, it seems nothing has changed.

If you love sweet romance stories that flourish against the odds, you'll love The Power of Will

The Letter

~Mary

Because love matters, differences don't.

ACKNOWLEDGMENTS

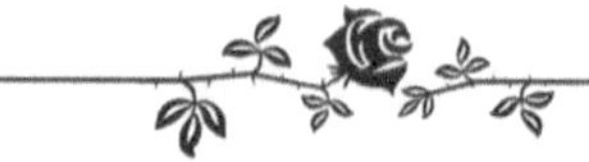

Writing a book like this is emotionally, physically and mentally challenging. Cancer is not an easy subject. Neither is wrongful conviction. Not every story has a happy ending. I tried my best to honor the real struggle people with cancer face while being honest about the emotions and the physical pain and suffering that accompanies such a battle. It's also difficult to be in the caretaker role of someone who is ill. It's important to recognize those people as well.

I want to thank all the brave people who shared their cancer stories with me — especially Patsy Brock Williams. Thank you for stepping forward and sharing information and encouraging us all to be proactive with our breast care.

I also want to thank fellow author, Tori Madison. I was about halfway through my book when I had a specific question about breast cancer treatment. During my research, I ran across Tori Madison's gripping books *Beneath It All* and *Beneath, Your Beautiful.* I highly recommend these phenomenal books. I binge read both of them in a single afternoon when I should've been writing. But beyond that, Tori took the time to answer my questions to make sure my book was as accurate as possible. I appreciate the support from another author — especially one who writes in my own genre.

My family has been incredibly helpful. My oldest son

is a doctor and he no longer even blinks when I ask him for imaginary diagnosis and treatment plans for characters which only exist in my head.

My youngest son has become a phenomenal proofreader and is quite adept at keeping me fed with delectable goodies like éclairs and homemade banana bread. Thank you so much for your help.

I could do none of this without the support of my husband Leonard. He is amazingly talented at fixing plotholes and un-twisting my ideas when I get stuck. I couldn't do this without your unabashed support I love you.

I talk a lot about the Girlfriend Posse in my books. But I have one of my own — Kathern Watts, Kathy Faltinson, Becca Draper-Ristanovic, Brianna Tubbs, and Lacie Redding, you guys are without a doubt the best. Thanks for always being in my corner.

ABOUT THE AUTHOR

I have been lucky enough to live my own version of a romance novel. I married the guy who kissed me at summer camp. He told me on the night we met that he was going to marry me and be the father of my children.

Eventually, I stopped giggling when he said it, and we've been married for more than thirty years. We have two children. The oldest is a Doctor of Osteopathy. He is across the United States completing his residency, but when he's done, he is going to come back to Oregon and practice Family Medicine. Our youngest son is now tackling high school and where he is an honor student. He is interested in becoming an EMT.

I write full time now. I have published more than thirty books and have several more underway. I volunteer my time to a variety of causes. I have worked as a Civil Rights Attorney and diversity advocate. I spent several years working for various social service agencies before becoming an attorney.

The Letter

In my spare time, I love to cook, decorate cakes and of course, I obsessively, compulsively read.

I would be honored if you would take a few moments out of your busy day to check out my website, MaryCrawfordAuthor.com. While you're there, you can sign up for my newsletter and get a free book. I will be announcing my upcoming books and giving sneak peeks as well as sponsoring giveaways and giving you information about other interesting events.

If you have questions or comments, please E-mail me at Mary@MaryCrawfordAuthor.com or find me on the following social networks:

Facebook: www.facebook.com/authormarycrawford

Website: MaryCrawfordAuthor.com

Twitter: www.twitter.com/MaryCrawfordAut

=